PRAISE FOR FRANK HUYLER'S *THE BLOOD OF STRANGERS*

"In lyrical and beautifully controlled prose, Frank Huyler takes us into the world of emergency medicine and in the process manages to leapfrog over all our preconceptions, erase all the stereotypes that television and movies have given us. This is a wonderful debut by a gifted writer and doctor."   —Abraham Verghese, author of
The Tennis Partner and *My Own Country*

"The author of these doctor stories is an E.R. physician as well as a poet, and his work shows the economy and sharp attention that both jobs demand."   —*The New Yorker*

"Dr. Huyler's short, intense book treats of only the most important matters: life and death. His prose is nearly invisible, and therefore it allows us to see what he is talking about. And once we see it, we are not likely to forget it. This is a young writer with a big mind—and an even bigger heart."   —Paul Auster, author of *Timbuktu*

"Moving . . . Huyler is a fine writer with an unerring eye for the dramatic metaphor. . . . What characterizes each of these miniatures is the candor in which they are offered, and their authenticity."
—Richard Selzer, *San Francisco Chronicle*

"A work of deep insight, whose tense prose echoes the sharp drama of the E.R."   —Jerome Groopman, M.D., author of
The Measure of Our Days and *Second Opinions*

"Huyler's writing is sharp and spare, clean as a scalpel....This volume is a modest jewel, a compact, faceted gem that shines with intelligence."
—Vicki Hengen, *The Boston Globe*

"If Raymond Carver had been a doctor, these are the stories he would have written. There are no untarnished heroes here. This is the world as it is: lovely and disturbing all at once."
—Atul Gawande, *New Yorker* staff writer

"Utterly engrossing, moving, poetic accounts."
—*Kirkus Reviews* (starred review)

"These bloods are so compassionately drawn, so eloquently examined, the results will stop your heart, and make you bleed for more."
—Joe Connelly, author of *Bringing Out the Dead*

"This haunting, exquisitely observed collection of medical vignettes is much more than a compilation of odd cases from the emergency room. Huyler probes beneath the surface to reveal the marrow of his encounters with patients . . . [inviting] the reader behind the drape."
—*Publishers Weekly* (starred review)

"Watch out! This book could make you miss your subway stop or an appointment. For Huyler is . . . a poet whose choice of words, conciseness, and feeling for rhythm draw one into the stories he tells."
—*Booklist*

"At times, Huyler's writing is so crisp and beautiful it startles. . . . His even-handed distribution of empathy brings to mind Chekhov and William Carlos Williams."
—David Kent, M.D.,
The New England Journal of Medicine

"Oh, the ability Huyler has to present the essence of common medical experience in transcendent, poetic prose, the stuff of the permanent memories of every doctor. Nonphysician readers will also appreciate the stories in their reality and their succinct and beautiful expression."
—*Journal of the American Medical Association*

The BLOOD of STRANGERS

The BLOOD of STRANGERS

STORIES FROM EMERGENCY MEDICINE

FRANK HUYLER

AN OWL BOOK
Henry Holt and Company | New York

Henry Holt and Company, LLC
Publishers since 1866
115 West 18th Street
New York, New York 10011

Henry Holt® is a registered trademark of
Henry Holt and Company, LLC.

Originally published in hardcover in 1999
by the University of California Press.

Library of Congress Cataloging-in-Publication Data
Huyler, Frank, date.
The blood of strangers: stories from emergency medicine /
Frank Huyler.—1st Owl Books ed.
p. cm.
Previously published: Berkeley: University of California Press, 1999.
ISBN 0-8050-6597-0 (pbk.)
1. Emergency medicine—Popular works. 2. Hospitals—
Emergency service—Popular works. I. Title.
RC87.H975 2000   00-027476
616.02'5—dc21

Henry Holt books are available for special promotions and
premiums. For details contact: Director, Special Markets.

First Owl Books Edition 2000

DESIGNED BY KELLY S. TOO

Printed in the United States of America
1   3   5   7   9   10   8   6   4   2

For my father and mother,
Frank and Marina Huyler

Contents

Acknowledgments

I am very grateful to the following people:

David Sklar, for his sustained enthusiasm and encouragement, without which this book would not have been possible.

Beth Hadas, for her invaluable assistance in finding a publisher for this book.

Helena Brandes, for her keen eye and her kindness.

Scott Huyler, for his sharp insight, his humor, and his constant support.

Kira Robinson, whose exacting standards prompted many revisions.

Holbrook Robinson, for his close and as always intelligent reading.

Chris Bannon, for his honesty, and his rigor.

Tim Steigenga, for his perceptive and kindhearted advice.

Thanks also to Peter Robinson, Scott Meskin, Tracy Hardister, Brent Jarrett, Wendy Johnson, Judith Brillman, Eugenia Perry, Jennifer MacGillvary, Johanna Sharp, Scott Graham, and Mike Howard, each of whom read various drafts of the manuscript and all of whose comments I valued greatly.

I would like to thank Nancy Jesser.

Lastly, thanks to Howard Boyer of the University of California Press for believing in this book, and Sarah Dry, also of UC Press, for shaping it into its finished form.

The BLOOD of STRANGERS

THE UNKNOWN ASSAILANT

ONE WAS MIDDLE-AGED, BALDING, THE OTHER YOUNG, OVER-weight, and both men screamed as they rolled in on the gurneys. We had no warning on the radio at all. The paramedics were urgent, moving quickly and breathing hard. Multiple gunshot wounds, they said, with unstable vital signs. They didn't have time to call it in; it was too close, they were too busy.

I took the young one. He lay soaked in sweat, with a blue-red hole in his neck. "I can't move my feet," he yelled, over and over. "I can't move my feet."

The volume of his shouts was like a physical force in the small space. We hung blood immediately—deep red, the icy drops tumbling into him as he grew quiet, and his face settled into the mottled blue mask I'd seen so often in that room.

On the X ray clipped to the board, the bullet appeared

magnified, white against the grays of his chest, just under his heart. As we ran to the operating room, the gurney humming like a shopping cart down the hall to the elevator, I heard the nurse on the phone behind me. "They're coming up right now," she said. "Get the room ready."

In the elevator, the slow minute of quiet, he looked up at me, and I felt his hand on mine. "Please," he said, like a small child beginning to cry, "I don't want to die. Don't let me die."

"You're not going to die," I replied, thinking he might very well. "We'll take care of you."

The bullet had clipped his aorta, torn through one lung, through the diaphragm, and into his belly. He lay on his side, his chest split open, while the surgeons struggled and cursed. With both hands I held his beating heart out of the way so the surgeons could see. His chest was like a misshapen bowl, dark and rich, filling again and again.

"Jesus Christ, this guy is making us work," Rosa, the surgery resident, said, scooping out handfuls of clotting blood which slid off the surgical drapes onto the floor. Sweat beaded up on her nose above the mask, then fell, drop by drop, into the wound.

There was so much blood they couldn't see what they were doing, putting in dozens of misplaced stitches until some began to stick, and the bleeding slowed to an ooze. He was cold by then, despite the anesthesiologist's best efforts and the heat turned all the way up in the room, his blood full of acid and losing its ability to clot.

"OK," Dr. Blake, the attending surgeon, said, "We've got to stop and just hope he doesn't break loose."

It was a long night in the ICU, transfusing him with unit after unit of blood and plasma. Toward morning he was no longer recognizable, swollen from the fluid, bruised, but miraculously alive. When I came to see him, before sunrise, I found a police officer sitting in a chair reading a magazine. The policeman yawned when he saw me, put down his magazine, and came out to talk.

"He's a bad one," he said, gesturing to the monstrously distorted figure. "We think he killed at least two convenience store clerks last year."

"Really?"

The cop nodded. "Killed them both, after he'd got the money." He made a shooting motion with thumb and forefinger. "Right through the head. We've been after him for a year."

I vaguely remembered the crime—front-page news, CONVENIENCE STORE CLERKS SHOT DEAD BY UNKNOWN ASSAILANT—and I looked at my patient as if for the first time. He didn't move at all, letting the machines do their work.

I learned the full story from the other wounded man. He was not my patient, but that morning I went to see him anyway. Ray Solano, lying down the hall, had been extraordinarily lucky.

He was wide awake, off the ventilator, and he looked up with a start when I came into the room. He'd been hit once in the chest, but somehow the bullet had followed a rib around and out the back without hitting any vital structures. He would be leaving the ICU shortly.

"Mr. Solano," I said. "I'm sorry to bother you so early. How are you feeling?"

"Alive," he replied, shaking his head, extending his hand. We shook, even though I'd done nothing for him.

"What happened?" The man looked at me, and I realized that he was going to cry.

"I knew he was going to do something as soon as he came into the store. He asked me for a job, and I told him I wasn't hiring." Mr. Solano looked up at the ceiling and took a deep breath. "Then he asked where my safe was, and I saw that he had a gun in his hand. I told him it was in the back, and then he just shot me. Right away, without asking anything else. I knew that he was going to shoot me again." He looked away, crying in earnest now, and I stopped asking questions, apologized, left his room.

The nurse filled me in. "He knew he was going to get shot again," she said, whispering. "That guy"—she gestured down the hall—"dragged him to the back, where the safe was, and told him to open it, and he went for the gun."

I imagined that struggle: middle-aged Ray Solano, already wounded, wrestling a much younger man, somehow turning the gun on his attacker and pulling the trigger, then staggering to the telephone. "There was blood all over the place," the cop had said, "like someone dragged it down the hall with a mop."

That night I saw my patient on TV. It was the lead story on the local news. A clip of the crime scene with ambulances, and then the smoky, black-and-white surveillance tapes of the previous murders: an overweight, unrecognizable figure standing in front of a cash register, his hand outstretched as if pointing at the men, then, very deliberately, two faint flashes, puffs of smoke, into their faces. They dropped like stones, the whole scene strange, distorted by the small wide-angle lens of the camera, like looking into a jar of water.

Over the next few days my patient began to wake up and was taken off the ventilator. I went to see him each morning, and he began to turn his head toward me, open his eyes. He started to look human again as the fluid eased out of him, his thick black hair flowing to the curve of his brown shoulders. He began to speak, to ask the nurse for ice, and within two days it was as if a light had come on; he was alert, back in the world.

"Thank you, sir," he said, intelligent, as I stood above him. "Thank you for saving my life."

"I didn't save your life," I replied. "The surgeons saved your life."

"That was you in the elevator, wasn't it?"

"Yes."

"I remember you."

Then later, quietly: "Do you think I'll be able to walk again?"

"I don't know. It's too early to tell."

He was unfailingly polite. He thanked me whenever I came into the room, speaking in a curiously childlike voice. I found myself drawn there, doing things for him: adjusting his pillows, bringing him a glass of water. There was an aura about him that fascinated me, a presence that the nurses also commented on. He seemed guiltless, unburdened by the act; his relief on learning that his victim was alive and would leave the hospital was real. It meant one less murder charge to face. The evidence of the others was not overwhelming, and he knew it. As did the police.

"That bastard might get off," one said, shaking his head. "It's a fucked-up world."

"Hello, Dr. Huyler," he said every morning, smiling at me, dark-eyed, his hair unkempt and thick against the pillows. There was knowledge there, and I was glad, even as weak as he was, that he meant me no harm, that I was not Mr. Solano, alone in the store and unready.

Each day I helped him get better.

The crow wished everything was black,
the owl that everything was white.

—WILLIAM BLAKE

PRELUDE

I HAD A 1972 MERCURY STATION WAGON WITH A CYLINDER gone, and at the end of that summer, when I left Boston for medical school in North Carolina, it pumped smoke all down the eastern seaboard, filling the rearview mirror with a blue haze. I felt like a slow rocket, sticking to the Naugahyde, sweat on my face, windows down, the back full of boxes and clothes.

It was one hundred degrees in New York, and on the Verrazano Narrows bridge, in a traffic jam, the needle rose off the top of the temperature gauge. On either side, the tenements, with men in undershirts at open windows, smoking cigarettes, still, looking down at the cars below. I turned on the heater full blast to cool the engine, and it must have been one hundred and twenty in the car. The world shimmered for a bit until at last the line began to move, and the sweet air came in through the windows, and I had chills.

I rented a small house at the edge of the college town, and I didn't own anything—an old car, a cat, a guitar, clothes, a few posters. The heavy, wet heat of the South, days in the dean's office, registering, writing my name, sitting still for the camera. In the evenings I made pasta and took it out with a beer to the porch, watching the thunderheads gather as my cat Tim rummaged in the dense undergrowth of the hill. After dark he brought home his mice and birds, like little wet clumps of cloth, and once he left a string of exact, bloody tracks across the linoleum floor of the kitchen to the couch in the living room. I was alone, I left them there for days, and when I finally cleaned them up the blood was dry, like powder.

The evening thunderstorms in Chapel Hill that summer seemed vast, beautiful, all deep bass and rain, and I lay in the dark listening to them. I would doze on the bed, then wake to more rain, and lightning, and water streaming out of the gutters off the roof. Then Tim would bang on the screen door with his paw until I got up to let him in, and he'd jump on the bed damp, purring, smelling like grass.

On the first day of anatomy, we stood in silence, staring at the bundle of greasy plastic on the gurney. My partner already had a black leather bag, a present from his family, with his name on the handle. He was small and dark, with brown hair and eyes, and he looked gentle. We wore new white lab coats, our hands did not yet smell of formalin, and I was trembling just a little, the fine hair on my arms rising in the air-conditioned cold of the room.

We introduced ourselves. "I'm Tony," he said. "It's nice to meet you." And the instructor unwrapped the body.

Our cadaver was sixty-two years old, and after a while, when we had gotten used to it, we cut around his tattoos and saved them, like a little pile of photographs which we left by his intact head. Mother. A red rose, and a woman's silhouette. The United States Navy.

When we reached it, the cancer in his lung felt like sand under the blade. I felt it in my hands long after the lesson was over. Foreign, gray like fog or gravel, there in the apex. It was strong and frightening, because even as we reduced him to pieces I knew that he was real, that he had stories to tell, that he had looked out at the sea from the decks of ships. I could feel it when I chose to. Mostly I chose not to. Mostly it was anatomy.

Three weeks later we carried his leg to the sink and washed the green stool out of the attached portion of his rectum. For the first time, it was too much, and I had to step outside, onto the high balcony. It was hot and still, and I held the railing, looking out over the pine forests that stretched for miles into the distance at the edge of town, knowing that I should go back inside. But I stood there anyway, emptying myself, until someone opened the door behind me.

"Are you OK?"

"I'm all right, Tony, thanks. I'll be there in a minute."

THROUGH THE DARK, SOFTLY

I COULDN'T BELIEVE WILLIAM WAS ALIVE. HE WAS LIKE someone out of the past, weary behind the barbed wire, blinking at the Allied soldiers at the gates. He was in his early forties, and all he did as he lay on the hospital bed was chew pieces of ice. After a while I came to identify that sound—the crunch of teeth on ice—with him. He was calm, alert, and he wanted only one thing now. This was why he was here, back home after all the years in Atlanta.

"Is there anything I can do for you?" I asked, after I shook his hand on the day we met. I was still a medical student then. I wouldn't be as open now.

"Yes," he said. "You can give me two hundred milligrams of morphine all at once."

In the silence that followed he smiled. "It's a joke," he said weakly, turning his head to look out the window.

It was springtime, with the dogwoods in bloom on the immaculate hospital grounds, and I often found him looking out at the gardens beyond the parking lot. Cars came and went, sun flooded the windows, nurses entered his room smelling of fresh air, and he lay quietly, watching all that life pour by and continue. In the late afternoon thunderheads gathered, and he looked forward, he said, to watching them.

His family didn't know what to make of him, what to do or say, but they came to see him anyway: his father and mother, in their mid-sixties, from a small town nearby, and his sister, strained, cheerful, who always wore office clothes. They sat by his bed, all three of them, and made small talk. Parties they'd been to. A wedding. The MacGregors selling their house and moving to Florida, who knew why. A card from the congregation, prayers from the neighbors across the street. "Oh, yes," he said. "I used to cut their lawn when I was a kid. That was nice of them."

Later, after they'd gone, he talked to me. Neither of us had much else to do that month. "My mother and father haven't really accepted that I'm dying," he said. "I just don't know what to say to them. They'll always remember it. I have to be so careful."

But it was impossible not to believe he was dying. His parents and I had discussed it. They wanted to know how long. "I really don't know," I said. "It could be a few weeks or it could be a few days. I'm sorry."

His father had started to cry then, and had tried to hide his tears from me. "My husband is an upstanding man," his wife said, after he left the room. "He's gone to church every Sunday his whole life. He prays for his son every night. He just doesn't understand why this is happening."

Later, his sister took me aside. "Mom and Dad don't really know why William left home for Atlanta," she said. "They couldn't understand why he wanted to drive a limousine in Atlanta instead of going to college. I couldn't tell them." She paused, looked away. "Or maybe underneath it they did know. I guess it doesn't really matter now." Then, after a silence: "Yesterday my mom said he looked exactly like Christ on the cross. It's true, don't you think?"

One afternoon, as I went into his room, a thunderstorm was raging outside, the kind of thunder you feel deep inside you, with lightning white through the window, wind whipping the tops of trees by the parking lot, and then the rain, a gray curtain sweeping over the cars until the window hummed with it, the gutters overhead like fountains.

"It's great, don't you think?" he said, turning to me, smiling, lost in the moment. "It's beautiful." A few people ran across the parking lot for the safety of their cars, and headlights came on along the far road. In a few minutes it was over, the sun shining again on the drying pools that littered the sidewalks and black asphalt.

"You know," he said, "when I was in Atlanta I saw this slide show by this famous performance artist. I forget his name. Anyway, he covered a parking lot with broken glass. It was at night, and he had all these fluorescent lights up, so they reflected off the glass. Do you know what I'm talking about?" I shook my head. "Well, he crawled across the parking lot. He was naked, and he crawled across a parking lot covered with glass. And then he had photographers take pictures of him. When he stood up he was covered with blood, only it looked black under the fluorescent lights. Do you know what he called the piece?" I shook my head again. " 'Through the Dark, Softly.' That was the name he gave it." He laughed.

"I was always sorry I never went to college," he said, after a little while. "But now I don't think that guy knew what he was talking about."

A few days later he decided to stop eating. No food, just water, morphine, and ice chips. What's the point, he said. It was the Friday before Memorial Day weekend, and I had three days off. I told him I'd see him when I got back.

He looked up at me. "Be careful driving, Frank," he said. "There are lots of accidents on Memorial Day weekend. I wouldn't want anything to happen. You have your whole future ahead of you."

I shook his hand, I thanked him, and just before I left I took him in my arms and lifted him to a more comfortable position on the pillows. He was too weak, too light, to move on his own, and I could pick him up without effort.

"You should probably wash your hands," he said when I was done, and I did, at the sink in the room, letting the surgical soap and hot water cover my hands and wrists, my bare forearms and elbows. The water felt good there.

As I walked to the door he stopped me again. "If I don't see you when you get back," he said, "thanks for everything you've done."

"I'll see you again, don't worry."

"No offense," he replied, "but I hope you don't."

And Tuesday morning, as I opened the door to his room, I could feel it. I knew what I would find. There was a figure on the bed. Beyond, through the window, the poplar trees dipped and swayed, full of sunlight and wind. As the door closed the figure sat up and turned toward me: a young man, his face handsome and full, with dark brown eyes, startled, as if woken suddenly from sleep.

"I'm sorry," I said, as I stood there staring at him. "I must have the wrong room."

FAITH

SHE WAS ANGRY, AND WOULDN'T LOOK AT ME, STARING INSTEAD out the window at the parking lot. It was hot already, in the late summer morning, and sparrows gathered at the feeder just outside her room.

"I want Pete," she said, as she watched them. Pete was a medical student who had recently rotated off the service. I was his replacement, a fact Mrs. Smith digested with visible regret.

"Mrs. Smith," I said, "I really think you should let us give you the blood thinner." She stared out the window. "Mrs. Smith?"

"The Lord knows more than you," she said curtly. "And I want you to leave me alone."

"Will you at least let me examine you?" She pondered. After a minute or so she nodded her head, almost imperceptibly.

I put my stethoscope, as I'd been taught, under her gown.

Her body was warm, stiff, and angry. I listened to her heart, steady and normal, and then to her lungs as she breathed. She was a young woman.

Bedridden for months now because of a back injury, she'd been having chest pain and shortness of breath. We knew that blood clots from her legs were rising into her lungs. Each day the attending, a lay Baptist minister, sat in her room quoting scripture and trying to convince her of the value of blood thinners. But she adamantly refused.

"I'll stand on the Word," she said, determined, looking straight into our eyes. "My faith is strong. Very strong."

When we entered the room, it was as if a light turned on inside her, a palpable hatred. I could understand her anger, I told myself, I could understand that we were all white men, with commands and judgment, but nonetheless I didn't understand a faith that required such risk, such renunciation. She whispered to herself, all the time, and it frightened me.

The Lord is my shepherd; I shall not want. He maketh me to lie down in green pastures: He leadeth me beside the still waters . . .

"The Lord helps those who help themselves," I said, but she kept whispering.

Yea, though I walk through the valley of the shadow of death, I will fear no evil . . .

"Did you hear me, Mrs. Smith? The Lord helps those who help themselves."

She sighed and stopped her prayers. "The Lord says forgive them," she said, "for they know not what they do."

It happened mid-sentence, shortly after lunch. She looked wide-eyed into the space over our heads and clawed briefly at the sheet with her left hand. Her body convulsed once, twice, then stopped moving.

The room was suddenly full of strangers and movement, voices shouting orders and voices shouting for quiet, the residents and nurses around me out of breath from running upstairs, the whole of it somehow detached from her still figure on the bed. The rituals of the code—oxygen, chest compressions, needles, shocks that convulsed her arms loosely off the sheet—had no effect. She just lay there, and after a while they stopped. As the crowd filed out, I stared at her. She looked undamaged, curiously undead, though not alive. She lacked the absolute pallor that dead white people have.

Later that afternoon, before we went home, the attending called us together. "I've just spoken to the pathologist," he said. "Let's go down and see what he found."

The morgue had windows, and sunlight filled the quiet room. The pathologist, a smiling bald man in an immaculate white coat, sat at his desk in the corner doing paperwork. The desk was the kind you might find in any office, with a hand-carved wooden nameplate, pens, photographs.

The body lay in the middle of the room on a stainless steel table. As I looked at it, naked, heavy, I saw that the top of the skull had been removed, like an egg, and the brain was gone. The head rested on a red rubber brick. The scalp was peeled forward off the skull, a red mask that covered the face. The torso was split down the middle, and the chest, like the head, was an empty vessel.

The organs lay in a cool pile on a steel counter. Heart, lungs, and stomach had been cut away in a single mass so that they could be lifted together by the trachea.

I don't know why I did this. I put on a pair of gloves, walked over to her, and pulled the scalp up, letting the skin of her forehead dangle into her skull case. And suddenly there she was, the woman who had said "I want Pete," the face which had looked so angry and alive out over the parking lot only a few hours before. Now I could have read anything there.

"It must have been the Word," the attending said, looking down at her, his face grim. For an instant he looked angry, vengeful.

And there it was, blue-black, the full size of my thumb, held in the pathologist's tweezers. The blood clot.

"Would any of you mind if I said a prayer?" The attending looked solemn, stern, but the anger I had seen was gone. Surprised, we simply nodded as he bowed his head and spoke.

Our father who art in heaven
Hallowed be Thy name.
Thy kingdom come, Thy will be done
on earth as it is in Heaven.
Give us this day our daily bread
and forgive us our trespasses
as we forgive those who trespass against us.
Lead us not into temptation
but deliver us from evil
for Thine is the kingdom, and the power
and the glory forever.

We all said Amen, and he lifted his head, opened his eyes. He looked calm and excited. There was a silence until the pathologist, an uneasy witness, cleared his throat.

"Well," he said. "I should really get back to it."

BLACK BAG

IN THE MIDDLE OF OUR THIRD YEAR, I FOUND HIM LEANING against the wall by the nurses' station. Tony, my first-year anatomy partner. It was well past midnight, both of us were on call, and he looked distraught, unshaven, in wrinkled scrubs and the stained short white coat we all wore. That afternoon one of the attendings had told him she was going to fail him for the month, that he would have to repeat his rotation.

"I keep falling asleep when she lectures to us in the conference room," he said, shaking his head. "I can't stay awake. She doesn't believe me." I wasn't sure what to say. "I haven't been able to sleep for weeks. My roommate always wakes me up."

"Why?"

"It's a long story," he said, looking down at the floor. "I don't want to go into it."

"Maybe you should move out."

"That's what Vance says." He looked up at me, then stretched his arms over his head, took a deep breath. "Maybe I will."

I knew what it was like to be exhausted. After lunch, postcall, through the drone of pancreatitis or renal failure, the military ache in your body. You watched your hand below you on the legal pad, and you thought about sleep. So I touched him on the shoulder, said a few words, and left him. He had not moved by the time I turned the corner of the long hallway.

A few days later I passed the conference room. The medicine attending stood at the board lecturing. Vance and Tony sat in the back. Vance took notes and listened, but Tony leaned against the wall, his face slack, his eyes closed. Every so often his head bobbed as the muscles in his neck relaxed, and he jerked awake. Then it started again.

It was not something she could accept. She failed him, and he had to repeat the month. I felt sorry for him—it seemed harsh, cruel, and we were all struggling. It was a world of super-ficial impressions, where an authoritative tone and firm demeanor went far, and most of us learned to be actors on rounds. Tony didn't get it, though. He continued to speak qui-etly, fumbling with papers and shifting from foot to foot, weak in the eyes of the judges.

I didn't know Vance well. He was tall and mild, reserved, with light red hair, and he spoke with a refined Southern accent. His father was a prominent cardiologist, as was his brother, but, like Tony, Vance struggled in class. They were not roommates, but they studied together all the time, and now they were on the same service. That afternoon, in the cafeteria, I asked him about Tony.

"Well," he said, in a tone that told me he would offer no details, "a lot is going on in his personal life. He'll be OK."

Several months later, on a Monday night in the ER, the woman rolled in screaming, tied to the gurney with thick, well-worn leather straps, like the kind found on good suitcases. She was in her fifties, cursing and spitting, twisting her thin white arms, arching her back. Her voice shot into the quiet, and everyone stood up, turned toward her. The paramedics were smiling, shaking their heads. She looked at them as if they were wild, her torturers, as if they were fire. She was well dressed, her graying hair carefully groomed.

The attending took me aside. "Guess who she is," he said. "Guess what she does for a living."

"I have no idea."

He looked left, then right, to make sure no one heard. "She's a full professor at the university. She's normally the nicest, most intelligent patient in the world. That's a hint." He paused. "What's your diagnosis, doctor?"

I looked at her. She lay still for an instant, and then the shrieks began again. "Well?"

"Psychiatric?"

"Be more specific."

"Mania?"

"Yes," he said. "Good. She's having an acute manic episode. She comes in about twice a year when her lithium level gets too low. Apparently she's very well known in her field."

"Should I see her?"

"Sure. We'll see her together."

The woman swore and slashed at the nurses with her short, manicured nails as they came to start the IV. By then her family had gathered, an older man, a young woman. They whispered to each other, and they looked weary.

"And what's this I heard," the attending said, as I reached for her chart, "about your classmate?"

I looked at him blankly.

"What about my classmate?"

"I was just at the faculty meeting. He murdered his roommate."

"He murdered his roommate? Who was it?"

"I can't remember his name. It was some kind of lovers' triangle."

I pressed him for details, but he didn't know any more. I reeled off a string of likely candidates, but he only shrugged. "The dean said it's going to be in the paper tomorrow. That's why I told you." He nodded at the chart in my hand. "Come on, there's work to do."

It was on the front page the next morning: MEDICAL STUDENT ARRESTED FOR MURDER. Beneath the headline, a photograph, a good likeness. Tony, my anatomy partner.

The story was brief: he was being held without bail in connection with the death of his roommate, with whom he was believed to have had an intimate relationship. The cause of death was lidocaine toxicity.

I hadn't even thought of Tony. He completely surprised me, and that night I saw him on TV, in leg irons, handcuffs, and a bright orange prison jumpsuit, unshaven, head bowed as they led him across the parking lot for the arraignment. He pleaded not guilty, and as the camera panned to his face I saw that he was crying. I stared at the screen for minutes, long after the newscaster had moved on to other stories. A cameo, that was it, the last time I saw him.

More details came out in the papers. He'd lived with the man for two years. The man had been involved with someone else, but he and Tony still lived together, still slept in the same room. The man suffered from migraine headaches, and Tony, with his black doctor's bag, had been treating him for months. He took Vistaril and Demerol and syringes from the hospital, injecting his friend when the headaches came. On the morning Tony called 911 the medics found a young man in a double bed, cold, with no mark on him.

The autopsy was a few days later, and Tony had asked to be present. He wanted to know what happened, he said.

We were all required to perform an autopsy during our second year. I can still see the man I autopsied, in his forties, black, eaten away by sickle-cell anemia, lying on the shining steel table. Dead for two days, hanging from a hook in the refrigerated locker, bloodless, waiting for the pathology resident to get to him. Despite the cold, when the pathologist cut into the man's abdomen the room immediately filled with the odor of decay. I had gagged, breathed slowly through the mask, gathering myself for the task at hand.

It must have been nearly the same. Tony, in the brightness of the top floor, where the windows opened out onto the flat green plains of North Carolina, standing in his white coat and mask, looking down at the still figure on the table, waiting, standing there as the dry incisions were made and the organs removed, as they were placed on the scales and noted in the ledger, as the odor filled the room.

But Tony had held that man in his arms, they had whispered together in the dark, and now he watched the interior emerge, the gathering and weighing, the blood sent in glass tubes to the lab. He must have known they suspected him. And later that afternoon, when the assays were complete and they knew, Tony simply went home to the apartment.

The police found empty bottles of lidocaine in Tony's black doctor's bag, in a closet. They had been watching him, as the days went by, and they had asked specifically for a lidocaine level, which was not part of a usual autopsy. Lidocaine—a local anesthetic, and a drug for treating dangerous rhythms in the heart. Either form is lethal in sufficient dose. The bottles are everywhere in the hospital.

What had it been?

I'm tired, Tony. I have a migraine again.

Do you want something for it?

I think so. You're working tonight.

Then the yellow rubber band on the arm, the vein rising up blue for the needle, and the needle going in, a little ball of clear fluid at the tip, then the band released and the plunger easing down. It had been dark in the room, Tony said in his statement. I came home to change, gave him some Vistaril for his migraine, and then I left.

Another night on call, X rays and blood to be gathered, cases to be learned and presented in the morning. Lying in the bunks of the call room with the others, looking up at the ceiling. Beepers going off, telephones dropped in the dark. Half-sleep. Bottles of Vistaril are a different shape from bottles of lidocaine, distinct to the hand.

They played the tapes on TV.

"911."

"Yes, my roommate, I think my roommate is dead. He's not breathing. I'm trying to give him CPR."

"Where are you located, sir?"

Tony wrote to Vance from his cell. "He says he's innocent," Vance said at lunch. "He says it was all an accident."

"Do you believe him?"

Vance looked down at his plate, thinking. "I'm not sure," he said, finally. "I don't think he really knows what happened. I think he was out of his mind."

And one day that spring, just before my residency began, I was waiting for the bus on the undergraduate campus. The woman stood a few feet away, waiting also, with a dark umbrella for the light rain that had just begun. At first I wasn't sure. But it was her. A man stood with her, perhaps a colleague, and they were speaking. As her bus came, and she folded her umbrella, shook the drops of water off it onto the dark pavement, I heard her voice.

"OK, then, I'll see you on Wednesday," she called, then disappeared up the steps into the bus.

She looked all the world like what she was, a professor, thin and angular, elegant in her black sweater and short gray hair, her glasses shiny with rain. The bus drove slowly away, and I wondered how she felt, knowing what she carried in her head. I wondered what her thoughts were like, if she could ever tell when the change was coming. I imagined her little bottle of lithium, kept in her purse like money. Lithium, molecular weight 6.9, number 3 on the periodic table of the elements. A pure substance, the only thing keeping her in the world. And she had no idea that I was watching.

A GOOD SCAR

HE WAS IN SO DEEP A COMA THAT I DIDN'T BOTHER USING local anesthetic when I sutured the wound in his face. It was Sunday afternoon in the ICU, and I had been called in from home to close the man's lacerations. The night before, on a dark road, he had gone through the windshield.

It was really a job for a plastic surgeon. The wound extended from the top of his scalp deep into the tissues around his eye, then down his cheek into his mouth. I knew why they had called me, the intern. The man was not expected to live.

I did my best, matching up the creases of his skin, easing the bright half-moon of the needle in and out, daubing away the dark blood that rose in little balls from the needle point, tying my knots like a fly fisherman. The thermostat in the room was turned up all the way, but he was cold—I could feel it through my gloves. After a while his face began to lose distinction to me. The wound stood out, became an entity unto itself. The earlier intimacy I had felt—bending over him as he lay there, my breath all around him—began to recede into the task.

It took hours, my back aching, my scrubs damp under my blue gown in the heat. The only sound was the regular hiss of the ventilator. The soft brown skin around his eye was like a child's; his eye looked straight up, the pupil never moving, even as I tented his eyelid, trying hard not to slip the point of the needle into the eye itself. When I'd finished, my hands shaking, I stopped, straightened, stepped away from the bed. He lay muffled in blankets, and it was only then that I saw, in the hollow between his knees, a single eagle feather and a small plastic bag full of yellow pollen, left by his family to save him.

The next morning I came back to check my work. His face looked whole; only the thin blue lines of nylon sutures betrayed the extent of his wound. It was only after at least a minute of admiring the job that I realized that the sound of the ventilator, my constant companion in the room the day before, was absent, and that the man was dead.

THE ENGINEER
IN THE DESERT

HE WAS IN HIS SIXTIES AND LAY GASPING FOR BREATH AS I walked into his room. I introduced myself, and he nodded, with effort. The nurse attached him to the cardiac monitor, fitted the oxygen cannula to his nose, started the IV.

"When did the pain start?" Early this morning. It had woken him up.

"Do you have any heart problems?" No.

"Do you have any other medical problems, like diabetes or high blood pressure?" He shook his head.

"Describe the pain for me. Is it sharp, or dull?" Dull, vague, in his chest, going up into his neck and down his left arm. He felt sick to his stomach. He felt like he couldn't breathe.

"Have you ever had this pain before?"

He looked up at me, breathing more easily now on the

oxygen, his lips growing pink again. "I had pain exactly like this thirty years ago," he said. "Probably before you were born. I'm a retired aeronautical engineer."

"That's a long time ago. I doubt it was related."

"Once you have it you don't forget it," he replied, and as we waited for the EKG he told me the story.

He was out in the desert, testing a new heat-seeking missile for the Air Force. The crew was up before dawn, and the target—burning oil drums—was visible for miles across the flats. He stood in the open with a radio, wearing a white dress shirt because he was expected at the office later that morning. They fired the missile from over the horizon, and it came across the desert at two thousand miles per hour. As the sun rose over the hills to the east, the missile lost course, wavering between the two sources of heat—the sun and the burning drums—before settling, by compromise, on the man in the desert. The brightness of his shirt, his body heat against the cold earth, were enough to draw the missile, and he saw it turn for him. He ran, slowly at first, then headlong, toward the trucks. They were hundreds of yards away. He realized there was no chance to reach them, or even a reason; nonetheless he ran, unable to breathe, his chest filling up, and just as suddenly the missile changed direction, flashing over him as it went back for the drums on the horizon. It was fifteen minutes before he collected himself, was able to walk back to the crowd.

Listening to him, I forgot the monitor lights, the nurse standing next to us. I imagined those slow seconds as he realized that he had become the target, that he had gone from detached observer, careful minion, to the prey itself, warm and alive, with all that speed bearing down on him. Then just as suddenly, the turn away, the flash over the burning target that meant redemption.

As he lay there in his crew cut and glasses, wires going into the thick gray hair on his chest, pale, beads of sweat clinging to his bare shoulders, I could picture him as a young man, clean in the 1960s, quick with numbers, smoking, with a dark thin tie. I could imagine his competence, his great distance, speaking coldly into radios, the voice of mission control—*the target is destroyed*.

And now this, and the voice was mine.

THE INVITATION

"HE'S HERE AGAIN," THE NURSE SAID, POINTING TO THE cubicle. "He's a hard one."

A thin man sat on the gurney at the heart station. He was shirtless and alert, like a sparrow, interested in the proceedings. A tech was attaching him to the cardiac monitor.

"Mr. Santana," I said, introducing myself, "what can I do for you?"

"I'm having chest pain," he replied. "And"—before I could ask—"it's a ten out of ten."

His silk shirt lay neatly folded on a chair. He wore a heavy silver necklace, dark with inlaid turquoise, and polished hand-woven cowboy boots, their tips emerging from his immaculate blue jeans like horns. He held his white cowboy hat, decorated with a single eagle feather, carefully in his lap.

He didn't look like someone having a heart attack. He looked like he was holding court. He smelled faintly of alcohol and cologne. Two large gray tufts of hair grew from his nipples. His chest looked owlish, wizened and wry, and he breathed without effort.

"You're beautiful," he said to the nurse, running a clean hand through his dyed jet-black hair. "You're lucky I'm old."

She shook her head at me. "Hold still, Mr. Santana. You're going to feel a big stick." And she slid the needle into one of the big ropy veins which rose from his wrist.

"Ooh, you're good," he said, smiling at me. "I didn't feel that at all."

"He's been here before," she told me. "And he always signs out against medical advice."

Mr. Santana had an abnormal EKG. "It's bad, isn't it?" he said, cheerfully rubbing his chest.

"How many heart attacks did you say you've had?"

"I've had three heart attacks, four heart surgeries, six cardiac catheterizations." He ticked them off on his thin brown fingers. "I smoke, I have high blood pressure, and once"—he paused, measuring the effect—"I was dead for four minutes."

"You were dead for four minutes?"

"Yes," he said. "And this hospital saved my life. I owe my life to you." He looked pleased.

"Mr. Santana, I need to go look at your chart. They're getting it from medical records now."

"I understand. You're young, you need to learn. I remember when I was your age. I had the world in the palm of my hand."

He held his cupped palm out for inspection. I looked at it for an instant, then turned to leave, but he stopped me. "Bury me in the Pecos," he said, suddenly earnest.

"What did you say?"

"I have a house in the Pecos wilderness, with two hundred acres. It's been in my family for over a hundred years. I want you to bury me there."

"You're not going to die, Mr. Santana. I don't think you're having a heart attack."

He wasn't listening. "It's real adobe, you know, very rare. The walls are four feet thick. One candle will keep it warm in winter. One candle"—he held up a finger—"that's all you need."

He had not been lying about his heart. The chart lay in volumes on the table in front of me, chronicling his journeys: three heart attacks, four heart surgeries, six cardiac catheterizations, and one note describing, in cryptic clinical jargon, a period of asystole lasting approximately four minutes. His heart had stopped on the table, and then, after the drugs and CPR, had come back.

The nurse was also right. There were dozens of ER visits, each with a signed release form saying he was leaving against medical advice. His signature was flowery, ornate, and practiced.

When I came back to his room I found him carefully buttoning his shirt, his fingers deft on the mother-of-pearl buttons. Monitor wires lay tangled on the bed.

"Mr. Santana," I said, "I think we should keep you in the hospital overnight. You could be having a heart attack."

"I'm always having a heart attack," he replied. "You didn't believe me, did you?"

"I believed you," I lied, "but I needed to make sure exactly what was done."

"And now you want me to stay?"

"Yes, I do."

He shook his head, chuckling, and smoothed his hair before delicately lowering his cowboy hat onto his head. "No, I think I'll be going. How old are you, anyway?"

"I'm twenty-eight."

"You've got a lot to learn, I can tell. No offense, I like you. Why don't you get me the against medical advice form."

The nurse came in to remove his IV and witness his signature. "Now if you'll be my nurse I'll stay," he said, winking at me. "I'd stay forever."

"I only work down here," she said, removing the needle.

He signed with a flourish, inclined his head to the nurse, and extended his hand to me. He shook firmly, as if we were completing a business transaction.

"It was a pleasure to meet you, young man. I hope you will be my doctor again."

"Thank you," I replied, not knowing exactly what to say. "Please come back if you change your mind."

"I'll tell you what. Come up to the Pecos with me. Bring your girlfriend. It's beautiful up there." And he handed me his card.

As I watched him walk vigorously off down the hall, head up, thin, I contemplated his invitation. I thought of his house in the Pecos, high in the spruce forest, with its four-foot-thick adobe walls, quiet, candlelit, warm in winter. I wouldn't go, but I knew that this strange invitation, given lightly, was somehow sincere, that he had offered me something for my trouble. The card was thick cream, with his name embossed in gold: J. Santana. Underneath was a phone number, and there was no address.

SUNDAY MORNING

WE HAD A FEW MINUTES OF CALM, WAITING IN OUR GOWNS and gloves, our heavy lead aprons, as the radio filled the trauma room. A pickup truck, high-speed rollover, two coming in. Teenagers.

The black boy, who came in first, was dead. He lay unmoving, eyes half open, with a clear plastic tube sticking out of his mouth, the paramedics still squeezing air into it through a blue rubber bag.

"He's in asystole," the paramedic said, meaning his heart was not beating. As I turned away, I noticed his hair, cascading to his shoulders, dark and shining, each strand braided and tied with red and green beads. It was the labor of hours.

The white boy was still alive, and the room changed for me; the silence on the far side, by the still gurney, instantly faded.

They wheeled him in, and it began: the IV needles into his arms, the sudden, astonishing red of the blood spilled from them on the floor, the monitor wires to his chest, voices rising, the room suddenly full of noise and speed.

He was blue, barely breathing. I took the laryngoscope, put the blade into his mouth, and immediately felt how deeply unconscious he was, how soft and unresisting the muscles were. I lifted his tongue and jaw and saw, very clearly, his vocal cords, a neat triangle, like two white glittering sticks. It was easy to pass the tube past them into his lungs. The oxygen flowed, and his face turned slowly pink, alive again. He was big and strong, with earrings in each ear, the sides of his head shaved, his brush cut dyed blond, curly and full of clotted blood.

It was only a few minutes later, after the X rays and calls to the blood bank, that I felt the back of his head. It was soft, and warm, and when I withdrew my hand it was covered with blood and gray tissue. The back of his head had been crushed. By that time I knew his name—John.

The clerk tapped me on the shoulder. "John's family is in the consultation room," she said. "Will you go talk to them?"

I knocked on the door, stepped inside. All eyes turned. "I'm sorry," I said, stiff, uneasy. "John is critically injured. The neurosurgeon is seeing him now."

"How bad is it?" the mother asked, half rising from her chair.

"It's bad," I said, "I'm sorry. I think you should be prepared for the worst."

She sat back down. "This isn't happening," she said to herself, softly. "This can't be happening."

"Is Keith dead?" the father asked. "We heard that Keith might be dead. Is that true?"

"Yes," I said. "Keith is dead."

The room erupted—life in the presence of great damage, the overweight, middle-aged mother standing to weep in her husband's arms, the husband looking into the distance over my shoulder, at the white hospital wall. In the corners, a younger brother and sister, still children, began to cry.

"I'm very sorry," I said, knowing that anything I might say to them now would be simply sounds from a great distance.

"He was staying with us," the father said. "He was John's best friend. They were driving back from the lake. They must have fallen asleep."

Then, later, "His family is in Colorado."

I nodded. John's father looked up at me. "Can I see Keith?" he asked.

He was perhaps forty, white, with long hair, tattoos on his arms, wearing a muscle shirt. As I led him back to the trauma room where Keith's body lay, I saw that goosebumps had risen on his arms and legs and he was shaking.

The room was clean, all of the earlier frenzy gone, blood mopped up, everything back in place. The nurses had covered Keith's body with clean sheets so that only his face was visible, the clear plastic tube still sticking out of his mouth, and the amazing luxuriance of his hair. He looked almost unharmed. I stood in the doorway and let the man approach on his own.

He walked up to the body and stood for long seconds. "This is him," he said. "This is really him."

He fumbled under the sheet for the boy's hand. Then he bent down, his long brown hair falling into the boy's face, and kissed him on the forehead.

It suddenly seemed very important that I look closely, as closely as I could, at this man taking on for the moment the role of the father to the dead son, kissing him softly, holding his hand, then turning back to me and the doorway.

THE SHORT ARM OF
CHROMOSOME 4

I LET HER SLEEP IT OFF IN THE HALL STRETCHER. SHE WAS blind drunk, and she stank, her light brown hair coiled on her neck, her blue eyes half open to the ceiling. She lay still, but every so often something happened: a twisting movement, a jerk on the gurney, one arm flailing into the air. Her lips trembled, and as I passed I could hear her muttering, fast and low, nonsensical.

She wore stained overalls and a bandanna. When the nurse took off her shoes her feet were black, crusted, and smelled so badly that we wrapped them in plastic bags. She lay under the IV fluids, her feet in shining plastic taped neatly at the ankle, and I left her there because she was nothing, really, another drunk on a warm summer night.

Early in the morning a man appeared. He wore a mechanic's blue shirt with "Bill" embroidered on the pocket. His hair was black and smooth, neatly combed, and he smelled of oil and cigarette smoke. He stood by her bed, looking down at her, and as I passed he touched my shoulder. "Excuse me," he asked, politely. "Can I talk to her doctor?" He gestured to the woman on the gurney.

"I'm her doctor."

"Can you tell me what's wrong with her?"

"She's drunk," I said. "That's all."

He nodded, as if expecting the answer. "I left her because of her drinking. She's my wife. She has Huntington's disease."

With that he stopped me. I looked at her chart again, and there, among the nurses' notes, barely legible, was written "Hutchinsons Disease?" She had told the triage nurse, or had tried to. "Huntington's disease?" I said.

I looked at her again, and suddenly it was clear—the twitching mouth, the spasmodic movements of the arms. I remembered the grainy film I had seen in medical school, shot in the 1950s, of patients with neurologic disorders. They were marched out for the camera to perform their dances, led across a room as the voice-over ran.

I had never seen a case of Huntington's disease, but I knew what it was: a genetic disorder that begins mysteriously in mid-life, progresses to insanity and death within a few years. The short arm of chromosome 4. She was near the end. She was also drunk.

"Can you get her to a room?"

His voice brought me back to the moment.

"Yes, of course," I mumbled. "Let me talk to the charge nurse."

The nurse moved her to a cubicle a few minutes later, but it was over an hour before I could get back to them. When I opened the curtain of the room I did not recognize the woman. She wore clean jeans and a T-shirt, new white socks. Her hair was damp and brushed. Someone had bathed her and dressed her, but no one was there.

I bent over to examine her again, and she was the same. No marks, no bruises, just the strong smell of alcohol, the incoherent mumbling, the episodic jerks of the arms. Nothing to be done but leave her until morning, when the social worker would come.

On my way out of the room I saw her husband again. He was coming back down the hall, holding a plastic bag full of reeking overalls and her shoes. A girl stood next to him. She was perhaps seventeen and quite beautiful, with long blond hair and blue eyes, taller than her father.

"This is our daughter," the man said to me. I looked at the girl. She looked back calmly, neither friendly nor unfriendly.

"Hello," I said. She nodded, then passed me and entered the cubicle, smelling of soap and faintly of perfume. She pulled the curtain.

They had done it together, father and daughter. They had taken off her clothes and washed her body and hair, in private. I realized that the new clothes must have been her daughter's, that for a few hours she had been remade into the image of wife and mother. I looked at the man, and he saw the question on my face.

"We don't know if our daughter has the gene," he said, looking down the hall. "She doesn't want to get tested."

When the girl emerged again I found myself staring at her. She was young or she was old. Her future would go on, or it would stop with her mother, whose muttering flowed out from under the curtain, a continuous low language which she, if the numbers aligned, would learn also.

NEEDLE

I WAS WALKING PAST X RAY ON MY WAY BACK TO THE emergency room. The door to one of the X-ray suites was open, and glancing inside I saw a surgery resident I knew peering anxiously at a patient's monitor. Even from the door I could see what it said: blood pressure 60/40. Heart rate 130.

"What's up?" I asked. The surgery resident turned.

"He's an MVA from the trauma room. We had to intubate him because he was so combative, but the CAT scan of his head and belly were normal. He's only got leg fractures—but his pressure just dropped."

The patient was a young man, heavily sedated, on the ventilator. He was very pale. There were three of us in the X-ray suite—the nurse, the surgery resident, and I—and in the half dark of the room we looked at each other. Something was happening. Stepping up to him, I put my stethoscope against his chest. Each mechanical breath filled his right lung, with a faint whooshing sound, like feathers brushed across a rough surface. His left lung, though, was nearly silent. As I listened the surgery resident opened the IV fluids wide, squeezing the bags in his hands to increase the flow.

"Let's get a chest X ray," I said. "He's already on the table, and his pressure just came up a bit."

We spent a few anxious moments, watching his blood pressure, waiting for the film to be developed. The X ray was still warm when we held it up to the light, and there it was: the left lung punctured, crumpled like a wet handkerchief, leaking air into the chest cavity, compressing the heart and the good lung. It was a classic, the kind that killed you in minutes: a tension pneumothorax.

I found myself sprinting down the hallway to the ER for a needle and syringe, fumbling in a drawer, turning, rushing back as patients and nurses stared at me. I felt like an actor in a melodrama, cutting around people with a needle in my hand, my white coat trailing behind me like a cape.

The man was ashen when I got to him, and I simply stuck the needle straight into his chest. Air hissed out of him like a bicycle tire, in little bubbles of bloody froth. I took the 60 cc syringe, attached it to the needle quivering between his ribs, and sucked. Then I detached the syringe, pushed the air out of it, and did it again—once, twice, four times, until the pull met resistance and the air was gone, the lung plump and full once more.

It was as dramatic an act as any I was likely to accomplish again, blood pressure rising to normal, heart rate falling to normal, all of us breathing hard. Almost as an afterthought I realized that I had saved him, that he was alive because of me.

Late that night, after my shift, I went to see him in the ICU. He was already off the ventilator and breathing on his own, waking up, coming back, making dim animal noises through a haze of morphine and Valium. I knew that he would leave whole, and I sat there in the dark for a while, watching the red and blue lights of the monitor, savoring him, taking something for myself.

THE DEAD LAKE

THE PAGERS WENT OFF HARSHLY, EARLY IN THE MORNING, and we stumbled out of our beds, waking up on the stairs as we went down to the ER. Gunshot wound to the head. A young woman.

She was there already, alive, trying to sit up on the gurney. She even spoke a few words: "I'm cold," and, a little later, "Where am I?"

She could move her arms and legs, but it was a terrible wound. A tiny hole, a splinter of bone just above her right ear, and I had to work my glove through the clot, rubbery and warm, to get to it. She spoke, and the hallway filled with her soft voice, all nonsense now, as we wheeled her to the CAT scanner.

The bullet had gone almost completely through her head.

The images rose, one after another, in cross-section on the screen: a visible track across the brain, like a finger through sugar spilled on a table. Bone fragments lit up, white against the gray background. By then Ruth, the neurosurgeon, was there, and she stared at the screen, stroking her chin.

"This is a potentially survivable injury," she said after a bit. "It's above the brainstem." Then she turned to me. "Ask the family about donor status, though. Just in case."

The family, as so many before them, sat in the consultation room. It's quiet, off the hall, clean, with two couches and a chair, and I've grown used to going into it. It's one of the rare moments when I feel powerful. Events emerge with my voice, families hang on my every word. A dark vanity, vaguely resisted. Speak the worst; they'll be happy if you're wrong.

"I'm Dr. Huyler," I said, as I've done many times. "Are you Kimberly's family?" They looked at me, an older man, a younger man. The rest were on the way. They wanted to know, and were terrified. I didn't look at them very closely. I might not have recognized them if I saw them on the street. I was tired, and the world was strange, seen from great distance.

"Please," the older man said. "Please tell me how bad it is."

"We'll know more in a few hours," I replied. "She's been shot in the head. It's a very serious injury, and I think you should be prepared for the worst."

It's my stock phrase: Be prepared for the worst. Not so brutal as the literal truth, but they knew what I meant.

"Is she going to surgery?"

"I don't think so. There's really nothing to operate on. The problem is that her brain is badly bruised and will start to swell.

We'll try to stop the swelling with medications, but they don't always work."

They looked down, nodding at their own feet. "Her fiancé shot her," the young man said. He was crying. "Then he went into the house and called 911. Then he shot himself."

"I know. The police told me." The fiancé was twenty. She was twenty-three. "First he did her," the cop had said. "Then he did himself."

I was the ICU resident, which meant that I was responsible for all of the patients in the surgical intensive care unit that night. So I stood by her for a few minutes before returning to the call room, watching Ruth shave the girl's head, check her landmarks—the edge of the eye, the bridge of the nose—then ease a foot-long needle into her scalp, through her skull, deep into her brain—a medieval act. The pressure monitor.

The call room was small, with bunk beds, a telephone, chipped white paint. An old television, a few posters, put up years ago: wintry Colorado mountains, palms in the Caribbean, and, over the couch, the one I looked at the most. A lake in New England, blue sky, a hill in the height of fall color, all golds and reds, down to the water's edge.

During those weeks I spent many hours in that room, waiting, trying to rest, expectant. Up for thirty-six hours, home to bed and deep, blind sleep for a night, then back on, again and again. A meditative state, after a while, dreamy, distant, alive with details: patients coming and going on gurneys, rhythms of lights and ventilators, numbers, pagers going off, stumbling awake, falling half asleep again. I lay in the dark with the male surgery residents, listening to them shift and snore in the bunks, all of us unshaven, our feet stinking in our tennis shoes. I felt empty and full. The girl stood out, though, she emerged from the background wholly formed, complete, like color on a white surface.

My family has a cabin in Vermont, by a lake, and it's the one place in my life I've always returned to. I'd lie on the torn couch looking at the poster and drift back to the familiar dirt roads of my childhood summers, the pastures opening on the way to the Mt. Holly General Store, where we bought milk and ice cream and bait. The bloodworms came in Styrofoam cups, with black earth, and lived for weeks in the refrigerator.

Early evening was the best time. My brother and I cast out with makeshift poles, sticks with lines attached, into the deep pools behind the rocks. It was our lake, full of fish, and it was alive. There are photographs of me there, as a small boy by the water with a fishing pole, and earlier, as an infant, naked on the beach. I remember how expectant we were, the worm easing down by the rock into the shadows. We wanted something to happen, we wanted it to come gliding out to us, miraculous, powerful, full of wonder.

Early that morning, around five, the nurse paged me. "I think she's brain-dead," he said. "Why don't you come and look?" Her blood pressure, her heart rate, her oxygen saturation—all were unchanged. The room was dark, but the day was starting: surgery residents coming in, nurses getting ready for shift change in two hours.

"What's her intercranial pressure?"

"In the eighties." Her brain was swelling uncontrollably, cutting off its own blood supply.

"Give her another fifty grams of mannitol," I said. "And let's increase her respiratory rate to thirty." Nearly useless steps. I bent over her, brushed the ventilator tubing aside, and lifted her eyelids. Even in the half dark I didn't need a flashlight. I could see it: one pupil dilated wide, complete, and the other small, pinpoint. Her swollen brain had compressed her brainstem, crushing the small nerves that open and close our pupils. She was dead now, though you wouldn't have known it to look at her.

"Have you called the neurosurgeons?"

He rolled his eyes. "I've been calling them for hours. They haven't done anything."

The neurosurgeons were on rounds, and I could see them, a cluster of white coats down the long hall. As I walked toward them their voices drifted out of the background and grew intelligible.

"I'm sorry to interrupt," I said, "but the patient in six is brain-dead." They shrugged their shoulders; they knew all about it.

"We need to make her a donor," Ruth replied. "I'll talk to the family this morning."

So now it was her organs we were taking care of. She was the best of donors, young, strong, undamaged in every other way, with decades left in her heart and lungs and kidneys, in her eyes and liver. A young woman in her prime. A good match.

There wasn't much to do. Her brain was dead, but her heart kept working in the dark anyway, her kidneys kept on making urine. She lay there like a person, she looked and smelled alive.

That morning there were pictures in her room. A family

portrait. A child on the grass. A girl in a white dress, smiling in the kitchen. She looked happy, excited. I've often seen these photographs. It's the nurses who do it. They tell the family, bring pictures, it will help us see her for what she is. Something that doesn't occur to us, the doctors, very often. Gestures, a curative power—this is why we are here, this is what we are working for. And I recognized the man in the photograph after all. He stood behind the girl, his hair still dark. Her father, whom I had spoken with in the consultation room.

Early that afternoon, as I could feel myself fading, wanting sleep more than anything, a new patient came into the ICU. I had to do a quick history and physical before I could go home.

Just back from the operating room, Mr. Griego lay a few doors down. He was awake, nearly alert. He spoke only Spanish. A few days earlier he'd tried to kill himself. He'd taken a deer rifle and put the barrel inside his mouth. At the last second, just as he pulled the trigger, he'd flinched, tried to turn away. The bullet had torn off his jaw, and he had wandered bleeding into the street, drunk, until a neighbor saw him. He was close to my age.

They'd operated all day, excising a piece of his shoulder blade, with muscle still attached, to make a crude new jaw. They shaped the bone, wired it to the base of his skull, and, for hours through a microscope, knit its small blood vessels to his carotid artery. They tried to fashion a new mouth, they tried to make him lips. In a sense they succeeded.

On the new chin were a half-dozen leeches, stuck there like small black swollen fingers. He couldn't see them or feel them, but the leeches were important. They drained congested blood from his chin, allowing it to grow. It remained pink as long as the leeches did their work. They would swell up, drop into the bandages, and gradually the chin would darken, turn dusky until the nurse reached into the jar for more, held them delicately with tweezers until they latched on. And then the chin bloomed.

"They cost six dollars each," the nurse said, holding the jar out to me. "They have to be kept in a special solution." I lifted the jar up to the light, and there were dozens of them, brown-black, curling around each other in the tan fluid, hungry and dissatisfied. He would use them all.

I had seen them only once before, the day we hiked to Tiny Pond, a small lake a few miles from our summer house. "There are no fish in this lake," my grandfather said as we arrived. "There is too much algae in the water, and it consumes the oxygen. But it should be fine to swim in."

The brown water stretched a quarter mile to the woods on the far shore. No houses, no sign of the human world, just my grandfather, my brother, and I, hot and sweaty, entering the cool water, swimming out past the shallows.

They were painless, and it took us a while to notice them: three or four on each of us, small things on our backs, on my grandfather's thigh. We rushed out of the water plucking them off. They left little bloody rings on our white skin, watery, oozing for long minutes. The lake changed for me then, became repugnant, exciting under the blue sky, with the easy slap of lake waves on the rocks, and the faint lake smell.

My brother picked up one of the leeches, put it on a fallen birch log, and began pounding it with a rock. At the first blow, blood splashed on the white bark. But the leech was resilient, like a piece of gristle. He struck it again and again, and it kept coiling back on itself, writhing on the log. When he was finally done he'd ground it to a paste, the blood dark now, an unrecognizable fluid.

When I came back to the ICU the next morning, rested from a night in my own bed, Kimberly was gone. Her room was empty, the photographs taken down. "They took her a few hours ago," the nurse said. "There was a transplant."

That evening, after hours of surgery, the transplant team came in through the door of the ICU: the anesthesiologists, the surgeons, and nurses, wheeling the man on the gurney. He was slack-faced, soft, with yellow folds of skin. A man in his fifties, his liver destroyed by alcohol. I knew what he would do to me. He would keep me up all night, transfusing him, following his urine output, the new liver fresh in its damaged bed. A transplant patient, and me here again to watch him, to wait for him to wake up, to come back changed and remade.

I don't know why it took me so long to realize who he was. He'd gotten Kimberly's liver. The liver was hers, and now I was charged with it again, watching the numbers emerge from the computer, her liver in his body at work, making his blood clot, his systems move once more. I had imagined her organs scattered across a dozen distant states, like ashes, but here she was.

During the night we slowed his IV drips, gave him blood and platelets. He opened his eyes, began to move his arms and legs, and by mid-morning the surgeons were pleased. He was doing well. "He'll be out of the unit tomorrow," they said, smiling at the bedside. "He's doing great."

His wife came to see him. Mrs. Wilson, as she introduced herself, looked old, much older than she was, smelling of cigarette smoke, with wrinkled brown skin and jet-black hair. She trembled as she held her husband's hand.

"I want to thank you all," she said, for perhaps the twentieth time. "I want to thank you for what you've done." Her hand on my arm was fierce, and she tried to pour herself into me with her gaze. I would do anything, it said, anything, and I found myself easing away from her, because all I could think about was his years of drinking, the blind nights of beer and Jack Daniels. I saw him drinking as a young man in the morning, as a ghostly figure in the background of those childhood photographs, as an uninvited guest. I imagined him with the child on the grass, and in the kitchen, with the girl, waiting, and then the young man on the telephone, the ambulance, her soft voice in the hall on the way to the CAT scanner. Finally it had come to this: a body on the bed, drifting up to the surface, nearly there.

And I went back to the call room, lay down on the couch again.

What flows out from behind the rock, what opens its mouth in the water and rises . . .

I need sleep, I told myself. I need to get it while I can.

My brother as a boy, standing on the rock, intent on the task, mayflies starring the surface of the still lake . . .

Go to sleep. They're going to call you soon. Close your eyes.

Then the pager, loud on my hip as I lay with the lights out. "This is Dr. Huyler. I was paged?"

"I need transfer orders for Mr. Griego. The plastic surgeons want to move him to the floor."

"All right. I'll be there in a minute."

I kept lying on the couch, staring at the ceiling, gathering myself. I didn't want to see Griego again, to go into his room and ask him how he was doing, to watch him nod and point. He could wait, but I wanted to be rid of him. So I got up, ran my fingers through my tangled hair, walked the short distance to his room.

He looked up at me. His new chin was pink. The leeches, their work done, lay bloated and dead in a bottle of pure alcohol. He couldn't speak, he couldn't smile or frown, but he watched me intently. The wounds on his face looked clean and terrible, and I thought of how he would scare his little daughter, whose picture rested on the nightstand.

"Bueno," I said finally. "You can go."

THE PRISONER

"WHY DON'T WE PLAN ON WITHDRAWING SUPPORT TONIGHT," the attending said, to settle the matter. "We'll give his sister time to get here." The sister was already driving, the family said, south from Colorado. She understood the urgency. The rest of the family had gathered for days, shuffling in to talk to him as he lay there on the ventilator. The guards were sick of them, bored, reading magazines in his room. It was protocol; all prisoners needed to be watched.

During the last few days of his life Mr. Garcia was watched all the time: by his family, by the prison guards, by nurses, by interns, and by me, the resident. He always looked the same: covered with tattoos, his arms pockmarked by years of shooting heroin and cocaine, his eyes half open to the ceiling, kept alive by the ventilator. On his chest, stretching from nipple to nipple, was the green figure of the Virgin Mary, her hands pressed together in prayer.

He was in for murder. Forty-five years old, with an abscess in his heart from shooting contaminated drugs into his veins, it had finally come to this: my shift, my night on call, my job to turn him off.

The attending tried to be gentle with the family. "There's really nothing more we can do," he said, predictably. "His heart is not working anymore, and he has abscesses all over his body, even in his brain." At some level they must have understood that their brother, father, and son was a drug addict and a murderer dying a slow death by his own hand, but that was not how they spoke of him. They talked reverently of the good life he had led, how he had suffered, how it was time to let him go, where he could rest in peace with the Lord. His daughters, young women with small children, cried, his mother cried, his brother shook his head, and the small waiting room outside the ICU filled with the sound of them long after we gravely shook their hands and left.

That night, tired as I was, their glib revision of him infuriated me. Their grief was real, but the words they used to describe it were not. It was a eulogy for another life, another man, a fiction, a wish. My anger was disproportionate, unseemly, I knew; but I was tired, I told myself, of staying up all night with bleeding alcoholics, overdosing drug addicts, murderers, and gang members, and I was tired of families who remade history for the convenience of personal loss. I was sick of giving my sleep and my thoughts to them.

But I did not want to turn Mr. Garcia off. The sister arrived, and the time came. The family crowded into the room, paying their last respects with Father Rivera, whose absolution I could hear as I waited outside. The attendings and residents from the day shift had gone. I had been left to do the job alone.

I leaned against the wall. My hands were shaking and weak where they rested on my thighs. I felt breathless and light-headed. By morning the man had to be dead. Otherwise there would be questions about costs and staffing, questions about me. It had to be done, but I put it off anyway. I checked on the other patients, called the laboratory, called my girlfriend. I would do it. He was hopeless, it was better for him, I wouldn't want that for myself, it wouldn't make any difference in the long run, he was expensive. Still an hour passed. Finally his nurse came up to me.

"I've drawn up two hundred milligrams of morphine," she said. "The family is in the waiting room."

The guard watched with interest. "How long do you think he'll last?" he asked.

"I don't know," I said. "It's possible that he'll live for quite a while."

He was unchanged, lying still in the bed, exactly as he had been for the past weeks when we had been trying to save him. "Should I start the morphine?" the nurse asked.

I nodded. "Give him a fifty milligram bolus."

She pushed the syringe, and nothing seemed to happen. We waited a few minutes. The guard was rapt. "OK," I said. "Extubate him." She disconnected the ventilator, hit the button to silence the automatic alarms, and pulled the tube out of his mouth.

At first nothing happened. Then faintly he began to gasp for breath, his mouth forming a dark circle. "Give him some more," I said, and she did. The gasping slowed, eased by the morphine, and finally stopped. His heart was a different matter; it kept going, in strong, regular blips on the monitor, on and on for minutes until finally it too began to weaken. Strange rhythms appeared, a whole language written in the jumping green light: sinus bradycardia, idioventricular bradycardia, ventricular tachycardia, sinus bradycardia again, ventricular fibrillation, then astonishingly normal beats, more fibrillation, and finally the flat, faintly undulating line, unreeling for long minutes as we watched him.

His family met me at the door.

"He didn't suffer at all," I said. "It was very peaceful."

They agreed with me.

NUMBERS AND VOICES

HIS PAGER TOOK BOTH NUMBERS AND VOICES. IT WAS A little black card on his hip, with a green diode and a screen. It weighed almost nothing, and could vibrate or ring. He wore it all the time. The world entered him through it.

"Whatcha got, slick?" he would say into the phone, and we'd tell him, and he would get into his truck and come in. His voice was the army and west Texas, a cracker from a rough town, sly, amused, full of dark things—surgery, for example, and the blues.

Dr. Blake was the head of the trauma service. He was a short, thin man, with slick hair and a razor part. He looked remarkably like Lee Harvey Oswald. I couldn't have guessed his age. When he wasn't working he would run for miles, ten, fifteen, twenty, in the hills outside the city. He was tireless.

He lived alone, in a small apartment. No one seemed to know much about his past life, and he didn't share, but one night I saw him in a bar. The band was playing behind me as I sipped my beer. When the lead guitarist started the solo, I turned around to watch, and it was him. I was sure of it. Over the glitter of bottles and the crowd, he stood on the edge of the stage with his eyes closed, his head thrown back. His fingers shivered on the neck, and he was good, he was passionate. I knew right away as I watched him that it was something true, that he loved it.

He was pleasant to the house staff, nodding, waiting for us to finish speaking on rounds, never interrupting. "Well," he'd say. "Why don't we bump up his TPN and come down a bit on the vent." Then we'd move on, and he would stand there, restless, arms folded, waiting for the next.

The nurses called him Ray, and he went through them like a thresher. There were many stories. The medical student who passed his office late one night, glanced in the window, saw them on top of his desk. I could imagine it, though I didn't want to: his scrubs down to his ankles, his bulging eyes and face, her legs around his waist.

"Whatcha got, slick?"

"Thirty-year-old rollover MVA, hemothorax on the right, intubated, grossly positive DPL. Chest tube is going in now, he's got two units hanging, pressure's around ninety systolic."

"I'll see ya." Click, a dial tone, it starts again.

Then the one who fainted when he broke it off, right there in the unit. "She went crazy," Rosa, the surgery resident, said. "She had an acute psychotic break right here and we had to restrain her. It was two months before she came back to work."

"He lives alone, doesn't he?"

"Yeah. But he told me once that he has two roommates: Stevie Ray Vaughan and Jack Daniels." She shook her head. "Notice how he looks hyperthyroid?"

"You're right, he does."

"That's because he is. He takes synthroid. I've heard him say how great it makes him feel. I'm telling you, he's nuts." And it explained a little: his tirelessness, his faintly bulging eyes, the slight tremor in his eyelids. The effects of excess thyroid hormone.

It didn't seem to matter what they looked like, or how old they were. The beautiful young physical therapist. The heavy, friendly clerk in her forties. I wondered what could have possessed him, and why those women had been drawn to him, with his sly west Texas accent and his agelessness, why they had gone so willingly into his office. They must have known how he used them up, that after a few months it would be over. But it didn't stop them. It was power, of course, and he was full of it.

He was full of many things. Synthroid, miles of empty roadsides, winter. And now her voice.

She began paging him. She bided her time until he was on rounds, with all of us there in the early morning. Vengeance.

"I'm in your office, Ray, I'm waiting for you."

Then his hand like a snake to the button on his hip.

"Let's fuck, Ray. I know you want to."

He stood there in front of everyone, shaking his head.

"I have something for you . . ."

She only did it a few times, knowing it would be enough, smiling and distant as she passed him in the hall. And he carried on, ignoring her because he had to. I never read anything on his face: no remorse, no anger, not even embarrassment. Just a slight narrowing of the eyes, a quick shake of the head. And a few days later he had another pager, one that took only numbers. By then it didn't matter.

On it went, during those last months I saw him. Rounds with Dr. Whistler. An unhealing wound on the belly, a vague odor, a thin green film on exposed muscle, the black threads of the sutures visible as the nurse pulled the packing free. "Looks like you mighta tied those knots a bit too tight, Dr. Whistler. She's about to split right open."

"Who knows what the incidence of wound dehiscence in diabetic patients is?" Dr. Whistler replied. "For a quarter?"

No one said anything, and Dr. Blake rocked back and forth on his heels. "Well, I didn't go to Harvard like you did but I believe it's about 15 percent"—he paused—"assuming good technique."

"It's 17 percent," Dr. Whistler replied, as their eyes met.

They were united against Dr. MacGregor. Dr. MacGregor was the chairman of surgery, grim, long-winded, given to the formal expression of rage. He was kind, but he didn't want you to know it. He would stand silently and watch them, looking much older than he was. And then, sooner or later, his face would grow pink, he would seem to swell, and we knew what was coming. Antibiotics again.

"I fail to understand," he would begin, enunciating precisely in his Alabama accent, "why anyone would see the utility of vancomycin in this patient. This is a goddamn travesty. Why do you think we have vancomycin-resistant enterococcus in this ICU? Do you people have any idea what you are doing to this man? You might as well take him out to the parking lot and shoot him in the head."

And MacGregor would continue, full of passion, about the inappropriate use of antibiotics in the surgical patient. We'd all heard it a dozen times, but only Dr. Blake would rock back on his heels, sigh, look contemptuously at the ceiling. Once he simply walked away, in the middle of rounds, without explanation.

He was helpless with himself.

"I'm not sure," Dr. MacGregor had said that day, as he looked impassively at Blake's retreating figure, "how much longer Dr. Blake will be with us."

He was not the kind to go quietly, and when it finally happened it was front-page news in the city paper: TRAUMA SURGEON SPEAKS OUT. And there he was, Blake in a white coat, looking forceful and clean, with quotes: "I could not in good conscience continue in the face of the substandard trauma care delivered to the people of this state."

And so he was gone. To Georgia, we heard. To another life, another hospital.

I'm waiting in your office, Ray . . .

"Everyone is entitled to their opinion," Dr. MacGregor responded in print. "However, we deliver and will continue to deliver the highest standard of care to the citizens of this state."

I know you want to . . .

"The thing about Ray," Rosa said afterward, "is that he was crazy."

No news, for a while. But then, months later, it did reach us. A new child, a new wife. A brief flurry of conversation on the unit, then telephone calls. "Did you hear?"

That was all he could muster, a little ripple, like a pebble cast into a still pool, the rings opening for the banks. That was it, and I could hear that radio conversation between the paramedics and the ER in my head. A few weeks ago now, two thousand miles to the east.

"Whatcha got?"

"Male, mid-forties, in the garage with the car on, cold, pulseless, fixed and dilated, no rhythm on the monitor. Looks like he's been here for hours. I'd like permission to call the code."

"All right, sounds reasonable."

Just like that, and I imagined him there, in his Georgia garage, drunk in his pickup as the engine filled him with exhaust and his face went slack against the door, the tape player flipping back and forth. And through it all his little daughter, safe in her crib a few rooms away.

Come downstairs, I have a surprise for you, I'm waiting . . .

Then his hand on the button, cutting it off, until his wife came home and found him.

A DIFFERENCE OF OPINION

"I DON'T THINK ANY OF US HERE SERIOUSLY EXPECT THIS man to survive," the attending said every morning when we reached room 6. We expected the remark. The intern would begin the presentation, and it was always the same.

"This is ICU day 28 for Mr. Johnson, a twenty-six-year-old cowboy with pneumonia, sepsis, respiratory failure, renal failure, and anemia . . ." A detailed analysis of each problem, in descending order of severity, then ensued. He was growing steadily worse. The ventilator had been at maximum settings for weeks, supplying the man's ruined lungs with just enough oxygen to ensure another identical presentation the next morning.

"This is ICU day 29 for Mr. Johnson . . ."

"I don't think any of us here seriously expect this man to

survive," the attending would say, and we would move on, halfway through rounds and already worn out.

Mr. Johnson was a bullrider, thrown at a local rodeo, who had broken several ribs. He'd gotten up, dusted himself off, gone home, and over a few days he had developed pneumonia in his injured lung. His family brought him in nearly unconscious, with both lungs full of pus, and over the ensuing weeks his other organs also failed: liver, kidneys, intestines. He lay drowning in his own fluid, the fever unrelenting, his family gathering and staring at him. Over the past few days they had stopped coming, consigning him, it seemed, to his fate alone.

One night, more than a month into his stay, I was on call when his blood pressure began dropping yet again. The intern and I stood looking at him, swollen like a toad on the ventilator. He always tormented us like this.

"Give him some more fluids," I said. "And let's go up on his dopamine." The nurse sighed; she'd heard all this before.

Listening to the ragged sounds of his lungs, I thought something had changed. His left lung sounded a bit quieter than it had the night before, an ominous sign. "All right," I said, resigned. "Let's get a chest X ray."

The chest X ray had not changed much. Looking hard, though, the radiology resident thought he saw a slight difference on the left. "Could be a pneumo," he said, "though I'm not sure. Let's get a CAT scan."

He referred to the possibility that air was leaking out of a hole in the lung, collapsing it. The treatment for this is minor surgery, done at the bedside. You cut into the chest between two ribs, insert a finger into the chest cavity, and push the lung out of the way. Then you slide a long plastic tube between the lung and the chest wall. When suction is applied through the tube, air and blood rush out, allowing the lung to re-expand. Mr. Johnson had been the victim of this procedure so often that his chest was a mass of wounds that refused to heal and oozed blood-tinged fluid into the bedding.

The intern and I looked at each other, shaking our heads. This meant hours of work, wheeling him with his ventilator and multiple IV drips down to the CAT scanner, waiting for the scan to be read, then putting in the chest tube and getting X rays to make sure we'd done it right. Any chance of sleeping that night vanished. It was already early morning, and we were tired.

"Looks like a pneumo, all right," the radiologist said, pointing to the dark mass of air visible on the CAT scan. "A pretty big one. I'm surprised we didn't see it better on the X ray."

Mr. Johnson's lung, by the time I finally cut down to it through the deep, soggy tissues of his chest wall, felt exactly like a piece of cork. It was stiff, as if already embalmed. "You've got to check this out," I said to the intern. "Put on some gloves and feel this thing."

For a few moments he felt around with his finger, then withdrew it, covered with blood, and held it instinctively up in the air. "Feels like a piece of meat," he said.

The next morning we were reprimanded. "I think we should seriously consider the ethics of performing such aggressive procedures in this man," the attending began. "I should have been called. It's high time, in fact, that we considered withdrawing support altogether."

There was a long silence. "He's a young guy," I protested. "And we've done it before. And it helped." This was only marginally true. His blood pressure had come up slightly, but it was hard to know why.

About this time another attending came on the service, and for the next few weeks he alternated call nights with his colleague. He had different views. "This is a young man," he would say, when we reached room 6. "This is exactly the kind of patient we should be most aggressive with."

A bizarre dynamic developed. On even days we did almost nothing, checked no lab work, stopped antibiotics and tube feeds, and nodded solemnly as the attending shook his head and said things like "The most important thing we can do now is keep this man comfortable."

On odd days it was the full-court press. We worked to undo the previous inactivity, checking arterial blood gases, blood cultures, and X rays, adding antibiotics and fluids, tinkering with the ventilator. We nodded solemnly as the attending said things like "This man deserves everything we can give him."

This went on for over a week, until my tenure in the ICU came to an end and I rotated back to the emergency room, leaving my nightly struggles with Mr. Johnson behind. I was glad; he had unfailingly robbed me of sleep, and I had come to dread him. I knew him intimately, had examined him dozens of times, turned him over to look at his back, put my gloved finger in his mouth, in his rectum, into the interior of his chest cavity, and I had never once exchanged a single word with him. He was gone from the waking world, as nearly dead as a human being can be, lying at the edge but never quite crossing over,

his body, his animal self just strong, or not strong, enough. I
had hoped many times that he would die.

About six months later I was walking down the long hall
back to the ER from the cafeteria. It was midafternoon, a slow
day. The door to the pulmonary clinic was open as I passed. A
few patients sat in plastic chairs, waiting for their appoint-
ments. In one corner, leaning casually against the wall, a man
stood reading a newspaper. The paper obscured his face, but as
he turned the page I saw it, and I stopped immediately. I felt a
strong and sudden force. It took me a few seconds; I knew the
man, I knew his face was significant, but I didn't know why.
Then I realized, disbelieving.

"Mr. Johnson?" I asked tentatively, stepping in through the
clinic door.

He looked up at me from his newspaper.

"Are you Mr. Johnson?" I asked, beginning to feel foolish.

"Yes," he said, looking at me suspiciously. "Do I know you?"

THE BLEEDING GIRL

MARIA WOULD NOT STOP BLEEDING. IT DEFINED HER NOW. She lay there, and it just went on, it wouldn't even slow down. Nothing we did, nothing we could think of, had any effect. She was a leaking vessel, day and night, and she was alert, watching as she filled up the bed.

A ritual developed. Every few hours I called the blood bank, and, expecting my call, they approved another transfusion for Maria. By the end of the week none of her own blood was left in her body. She was full of the blood of strangers.

The distance between Maria's room in the pediatric intensive care unit and the linen closet was only about thirty feet. An older man mopped the hall. He had gray hair, thick black glasses, and he wore a brown janitor's shirt with his name, José, embroidered on the shoulder. During normal times we rarely saw him, but over the past few days we had called him often.

Every three hours or so a nurse wearing a heavy cloth gown and gloves carried an armload of sheets from Maria's room to the linen closet, and every three hours José appeared, picked up the mop by the door, and carefully followed the nurse down the hall, mopping up the drops of blood that fell like dimes on the floor. After a while he left his mop and pail next to Maria's room because he was tired of carrying them up the stairs.

Maria's mother, a young, heavyset woman, initially so tearful and tentative, was no longer afraid. Her manner toward us had hardened; she barely acknowledged me when we met in the hall. By now she wanted the vigil over, wanted her daughter to die. She stood in the doorway and watched José as he painstakingly followed the nurse. When he had finished he put the bucket and mop back by the door and nodded to her. None of us knew what to say.

The girl had juvenile rheumatoid arthritis, and a few days earlier I had saved her life. It was the single best thing I had done in my residency.

It had begun with her bones, the joints of her fingers and toes, her elbows and knees and spine, fused, frozen beyond function. She could barely lift her arms, she could not turn her head or look up. Years of pills: prednisone, Cytoxan. Eighteen years old. She did not menstruate or walk. Her skin was as delicate as paper, with a fine tracery of blue veins which burst at the slightest touch of a needle.

It ended with her kidneys. Every two days we plugged her in, attached the dialysis machine to the plastic tube that emerged from her chest. Last year she had passed up the opportunity for a kidney transplant against the urging of her doctors and mother. She wanted to go to the prom.

On the second day of her hospitalization they paged me overhead to her room. She lay gasping, frothing at the mouth, black-eyed, desperate, her lungs full of fluid.

The attending and I stood by the bed and looked at each other.

"We need to intubate her," he said. "We need to do it right now." He got the equipment ready. We both knew it would be hard, maybe impossible. We would insert a dull metal blade into her mouth, attempt to lift her jaw and tongue away from her vocal cords, and insert a plastic tube into her trachea. We could breathe for her then, with a machine and pure oxygen. Without it she would die in a few minutes.

But her spine was a dry stick, her chin rigid against her chest. Her bones were as brittle as glass. Too much force on the blade would break her neck.

"I can't see anything," the attending said, his voice rising, forcing the blade into her mouth, trying to look into her throat. "I can't get it." She was blue, and there was no time left. I found myself running, a full sprint down the hall, the stairs, into the emergency room, where they kept special tubes, thinner and more pliable, designed to enter the trachea through the nose. Then back up the stairs, charging through the doors, down the hall to her bed.

He was still trying, white-faced, determined, but it was no good, and he stepped aside when he saw me. I bent over her, yelled for quiet, held my breath, and slowly slid the tube into her left nostril. In the stillness of the room, over my pounding heart, with my ear to the tube, I heard her at the other end. A faint whistle, inhaling. I waited, and when it came again I plunged the tube in, hoping it would go, hoping her weak effort would be enough, that she would suck the tube down into her lungs.

"You're in!" the attending said, listening with his stethoscope. And I was—her chest filled with oxygen, her face bloomed, she woke up. The attending turned, his hand strong on my shoulder. "That was a great job," he said. "A great job."

I felt wild and full that day, exultant. I'd saved her, I felt as though she were mine. She woke up. Her mother cried tears of joy and exhaustion and release, and even the nurses praised me. I was good, I thought then. I was a good doctor after all.

I passionately wanted her to live. I wanted to keep my act, I wanted it badly. So when she first started oozing from her IV sites, her mouth, her nose, sinking into it, tired but still afraid, watching herself go, I told myself it would stop. Just one more day, it will stop. It will slow down. It will let us catch up.

The ringing phone: "Blood bank."

"This is Dr. Huyler. We need four more units of blood for Maria Gonzales."

"OK, we're sending it up. But we're running low. We're going to have to send out for it soon."

And so the blood started coming in by air from California and Colorado. It arrived cold, a deep icy red, the plastic bags stacked in cardboard boxes, with labels: Biohazard.

She became the center of something. Airplanes converging, the whispering voices of consultants. Literature searches, abstracts of scientific papers inserted in the chart. The whir of machines, and she bled through it all.

When Maria's mother finally had enough, she spoke first to José. "Take the mop away," she said to him as he stood by the door. "You don't need it anymore."

So we stopped the transfusions, and six hours later Maria died. They wheeled her down the hall, covered by a clean sheet. We stood there, the attending and I, the nurses, not speaking. Her mother walked with her for a little while, composed and quiet, then paused, looking at her daughter's still figure before turning away down the stairs. She was done with us, and we did not see her again.

A few days later a friend invited me to his house for Passover. I had never been to a seder, and I sat awkwardly as he read in Hebrew, wondering about the significance of the horseradish, the parsley, the lamb bone in the center of the table. Before the meal, before the breaking of the matzoh, came a series of prayers—the plagues which had fallen on Egypt. After each prayer we dipped a finger in our wine glasses and touched our empty plates. As I looked down at my plate, it seemed to expand, to stretch out in all directions. It became vast, the drops of wine on the white surface leading away into the distance. Maria, I thought suddenly, the girl whose life I saved, who woke up again because of me. Maria, wheeled into the bright depths of the hall.

Then another toast, and another.

I'M DRIVING

THE MORGUE AT THE UNIVERSITY OF NEW MEXICO IS A STONE
building, squat, determined-looking, with a glass foyer. It keeps
strictly daylight hours. There are usually a few police cars out
front, cops standing around smoking and talking. You pass
them, enter the unlocked door, then speak into an intercom:
"I have an appointment . . . I'm here to see . . ." and they buzz
you in.

After a few visits the receptionist recognized my voice. "It's
Frank Huyler," I'd say, standing in the heat of the foyer, and he
would hit the button that opened the door. The receptionist
had extremely white teeth, a black beard, and wore ties with
hunting themes: waterfowl rising off the marshes, a buck in a
clearing, a hooked trout breaking the surface. A desk, soft car-
peting, a couch with magazines—*American Rifleman, Field &*

Stream—and a book to sign. I'd write my name and the date, clip the visitor tag to my shirt, and go to the back, where I had been given a temporary desk.

The rooms were offices, with coffee pots, computers, floral prints. I'd walk down the hall, turn left, sit at my desk, unpack my portable computer, and look at the stacks of legal-sized manila envelopes that lay there.

The envelopes were arranged by year. I was typing them into my computer, distilling them to a residue. I'd hit a button, the computer would whir for a few seconds, and I'd close the envelope, put it aside, and reach for the next. I could do one every six minutes.

First I looked at the date of birth and social security number. Then the police narrative, the description of the scene, interviews with family and friends. Then the notes and autopsy report, and finally the photographs.

In the beginning I looked at the photographs. Tucked neatly in a corner of the page, they were strong offerings—the image itself, the act done, the car in the garage, the ligature, the jumbled figure at the side of the bed, the woman in the woods.

The woman in the woods stopped me from looking at the photographs. She lay in a small clearing, a hundred yards from the trail. Her clothes, her running shoes, her bottle of Evian spring water all looked new, untouched by the weeks that had passed. There was a close-up of her revolver on pine needles, blue-black, a mahogany grip, a touch of rust on the barrel.

The body received is that of a middle-aged Caucasian woman in the advanced stages of . . .

The police, caught in the background of the Polaroids, held cloths over their mouths. The photographer had stepped right up, aimed the camera straight into it.

I worked automatically, daydreaming, sipping a cup of bitter coffee from the pot, shifting in my chair. The envelopes flowed past my fingers, another entry done, the hum of the disk drive, conversations half overheard between secretaries at the other end of the room: salsa dancing, husbands, the teenager on the basketball team. Then the outside world, leaving for the day, nodding at the receptionist, the cops outside, acquaintances in the parking lot as I walked home by the medical library, the Sandia mountains blue and dusted with snow, the clear abstract sky.

I found myself thinking of my grandmother, whom I never met; how she had gone into the garage and started the car, determined, and how what she did echoes through my family fifty years later. Her social security number. Rye, New York. Westchester County. Her beautiful face. Wartime. Glenn Miller at the Ritz, my grandfather's uniform.

The body received is that of a Caucasian woman appearing the stated age of 37 years . . .

Enough of that, I told myself. This is only a research project, a residency requirement. This is descriptive statistics, epidemiology, preventive medicine, the identification of risk. Intervention strategies will be developed . . . our data show that . . . here we see the trend in 1994 . . . the Native American population reveals an age distribution . . .

The sun really heats up the foyer, well over eighty degrees, like a greenhouse: amaryllis, hibiscus, tropics in winter.

Time to go home and save what I've done.

After a week I had to get out. I left early Saturday morning, driving toward the Manzano mountains. The air both warm and wintry, a few cars on the road, countryside. Spring already, I realized, with only a few patches of snow under the trees.

Just outside of the town of Chilili there was a strange, bright metal sign by the side of the road: Chilili Cemetery, next left. I had been driving awhile, stiff, and I pulled over almost without thinking, parked the car, and crossed the road to the cemetery gate.

The cemetery is surrounded by a barbed-wire fence. It is small, with brightly painted crosses, in blues and reds, and there are flowers. Looking over the fence, I saw metalwork everywhere: six-foot towers, dozens of glittering plaques. Wind blew through metal chimes. All the work of one man. He's made cages over the graves, erected crosses, hung mobiles, and finally tapped his name on a plaque by the gate: metalwork done by Horace MacAffee.

Horace MacAffee's relatives are everywhere in the place, and he has a vision. He takes galvanized steel plates and bangs names on them with a ballpeen hammer. Virgil MacAffee, Mary MacAffee, the child of Maureen MacAffee, September 1937. George MacAffee, April 1990. The Lord's Prayer, crude etchings of Mary and Joseph, the baby Jesus in the children's section.

This has been going on for years; some of the plaques are

bleached by the sun, have a hint of rust. An Anglo name, MacAffee, but that hasn't stopped him. He's done the Garcias, the Trujillos, and Lopezes. He made the gate at the front, a car door attached to a spring.

Strange acts, no clear purpose. What is he doing? I thought as I wandered through the graves. Why is he so determined?

There were a few bare mounds of dirt, with no crosses, and I wandered over to them. Three in a row. They were marked with plastic tags, like those used for luggage at airports. Names and dates. 1919–1994. Garcia Mortuary. 1906–1994. 1921–1994. Dead two years now.

But the graves were fresh. For some reason the bodies had been exhumed, moved, reburied. The tracks of the bulldozer were still visible on the ground.

I imagined Horace at work in his basement, tapping with his hammer, misspelling "ascended" again, as he'd done throughout the cemetery. Accended. The Epidemiology of Female Suicide in New Mexico.

Then there were the notes.

Why did I do it?

1. mom tells me to turn down the stereo and never tells Larry
2. Julie
3. mom always yells at me

The body received is that of an adult female appearing the stated age of 15 years . . .

OK, I thought as I drove on, I'm Horace MacAffee.

I'm really going to miss you guys . . .

Like going to camp for the summer. Like moving away.

Don't think about it, I told myself, you don't want to understand it.

Guns. Hundreds of them. Rossi, Smith & Wesson, Colt, Ruger, Glock, Browning, .22, .38, .45, 9 mm, hollowpoint, wadcutter, yellowjacket.

In conclusion, if we could limit the easy availability of firearms to these populations, we estimate that we . . .

A statistics professor of mine once said, "If you look at the world, you will find the normal distribution everywhere." If you take a population of stones in a riverbed, he went on, and weigh each one, you will find that some stones weigh a little, and that some stones weigh a lot, and that most are somewhere in the middle. If you plot their weights on a piece of paper you will get the normal distribution, the bell curve. Every single river in the world will give you the bell curve in its stones. This is because some stones are hard, and wear down slowly. Others are soft and wear down quickly. Most stones are somewhere in the middle.

I remember being captivated by his analogy: the stones of rivers, the leaves of trees, the speed of the flights of birds, all described by a single curve, the rough shape of a bell, the world in order. It had beauty in the way he put it, but he had deceived us, as he admitted the next semester. In many cases, he said, the normal distribution cannot be assumed. The curve looks different. There are many more grains of sand than boulders. It all depends on how you look, and where.

Her husband had looked for her all morning before finding the deceased approximately two miles from the residence in a heavily wooded area which she was known to have frequented.

I imagine Horace growing old, stopping his work. A curious legacy, and finally I reached her. The last woman of the year. A partial autopsy, one more note.

It was something I could imagine; a summer night, the car on the road, speed, windows down, bright lights—

I was perhaps three, with a high fever, and whenever my mother left the room the image reappeared. It was an enormous steam locomotive with a single light in front, coming slowly forward. On the tracks, curled in the fetal position, was a child—me. I could not move, could not get up, watching myself from a distance. The locomotive kept coming, and I screamed, and my mother entered my room, and when she did the image went away. When she went back to bed it returned. And so on till morning.

"I'm driving," the woman wrote. "Somewhere there will be a train."

BURN

THE MAN CAME BY AIR, SOUTH FROM THE COLORADO BORDER.
He was alert, asking for morphine and his wife. They wheeled
him directly from the helipad, under the roar of the blades,
down the hall to the tub room.

The tub room is always first. It's two hundred gallons, stainless steel, 98.6 degrees, antiseptic, with wisps of steam rising,
and a block and tackle above it. After a while, everyone lying
in the rooms beyond comes to fear it. They keep the morphine
in a locked chest nearby, in dozens of cold vials, and refill the
chest every week.

Over two years I had seen many people lowered into that
water by the pulley, old men and children, babies and young
women, all naked, held in the arms of the nurses as they floated
there, their eyes dreamy from the needle, trying to be still as

the bandages soaked through and were pulled away. And when they were done, wrapped in gauze again, the surface of the water was alive with dead skin, like white cellophane, as the tub drained. Then a nurse would climb in with bleach, wipe the metal bottom with a sponge, gather up the skin with the glove of her free hand, and squeeze the water out of it.

But he didn't know yet what it was like, and was calm as we lowered him in, peeled off the bandages. Sixty percent of his body, from the nipples down, a mass of blisters and white.

In the burn unit, pain is a good thing. It means the tissue is alive, that it will come back again. Blisters are fine, they are hope. But then there is the dead gray, like an eye, and when you touch it, when you push hard, there is no reaction in the face, no further blanch beneath the finger. This is a third-degree burn, which sears the nerves, and it is the kind that kills you. Though Mr. Stone was only fifty, and strong, we knew right away that it would be a near thing.

"It was a box canyon," he said, as he lay there in the water. "We thought we were somewhere else." He shook his head, looking at the ceiling. They had banked in, flying down the center, the walls pouring by on either side. They had rounded a bend, and suddenly saw it. The end of the canyon, rising a thousand feet above them, all red sandstone, coming up through the windshield. There was no room to turn, no time to climb out. And so they waited, throttle back, flaps down, drifting to the streambed and the trees at the base of the canyon wall.

"All I remember after that," he said, "was the fire." Dr. Whistler smiled and left the room.

Dr. Whistler was a tall man, thin, with curly brown hair going gray, and small gold-rimmed glasses. He looked intelligent and kind, and he was widely read. He had a degree in philosophy from Harvard, and he made sure we knew it. On rounds, he would decorate his remarks with literary quotations: Li Po, or Shakespeare. Once I called him on it.

"Quoting *Hamlet*, Dr. Whistler?"

"Act?" he shot back, assessing me.

"I don't know."

"Three," he said, with a little smile, before turning off down the hall. "Act three." He loved burns.

Day five was the first harvest day, and Dr. Whistler was ready. He stood in the room in his gown, razors waiting, and folded his arms as Mr. Stone rolled in. He'd made it this far alive. We'd poured a river of fluids into him by now, and he was a lucky man.

Burn surgery is simple. You take a straight razor to the burns and shave down through them until you are in live tissue, and blood rises, in a hundred tiny points, from the flat surface of the wound. You want a bed of severed capillaries, where blood can rise to the grafts.

But you also need good skin to graft, and Mr. Stone didn't have much left. We started with his shoulders, and his round, untouched back. This was my job.

I used an electric razor. There is some technique to it: finding the proper angle, the necessary flick of the wrist at the end of the streak. But when you do it right there is a curious pleasure there, the skin rising, curling up like a slice of cheese from the blade. When you're done you have a rectangular sheet of split skin about two inches wide and four inches long. When you do it right it is translucent.

But you also leave a mark, a matching bloody rectangle on the shoulder, a sign. And you have to let it heal, to let the skin grow back, before you can take it again. Mr. Stone didn't have enough good skin to cover all his burns, and so we waited, did this many times, the skin healing, machined away, coming back again. The labor of weeks.

The skin was precious, and we got the most out of it. We fed the sheets through the hole-puncher, and what emerged was like a fishnet stocking. It could be stretched now, like bad rubber, and this was what we used to cover him. We simply stapled it down to the bleeding bed, wrapped it tightly, hoped it would take.

"It's like slaughtering a hog," Dr. Whistler said happily. And it was true. It was hot, bloody work, the thermostat turned up all the way to keep Mr. Stone warm, since the air on his exposed tissue acted like a fan through a wet sheet. He could die of cold, and we had to be quick.

"Sorry, piggy," Dr. Whistler said, looking around to see if anyone caught the reference. Then he shook his head. "William Golding," he said. *"Lord of the Flies."*

When he was awake, Mr. Stone read *Flying* magazine in his room. "Don't tell my wife," he said, before tucking it away under his pillow.

"Are you really going to fly again?"

"It was just bad luck, stupidity," he replied. "If I'd been a little more careful with the map it never would have happened. I've learned my lesson."

"What's that?"

"You just have to be certain, that's all. You just have to know exactly where you are, and where you're going."

But Mr. Stone was in the burn unit, and he was going to the tub room.

I imagined what he must have felt, the cliff coming up like an acquaintance, deadly and quiet, and how the cockpit suddenly filled with details—dust on the yoke, an empty coffee cup. And then the fire, rising. Looking at him, he seemed miraculous, like a visitor to the world. And here he was, leafing calmly through the magazine. "Bonanza!" the cover read, and in the photograph the plane turned away gently over the green land.

"What's the most poisonous snake in the world?" Dr. Whistler demanded, peering at us through his small round glasses.

"The green mamba?"

"No," he said, triumphant. "That's on land. The most poisonous snake in the world is the fire snake. It's a sea snake."

He tapped the bridge of his nose, and I wondered why he knew that, and why he had displayed that knowledge.

Mr. Stone's wife was twenty years his junior, and she wanted a child. She stood by her husband's bed as he lay uncovered, his torso and legs, his genitals: all bluish-red leathery ridges, where the grafts grew. She held his hand, and she met with Dr. Whistler in private. The next day it was news. "He's going to try and reproduce," Dr. Whistler said gleefully on rounds, rocking back and forth on the balls of his feet.

On it went, the weeks flowing to months, Mr. Stone

skinned and reskinned in the hot room as Dr. Whistler stood there with his razor, wiping it briskly on his gown, cheerful, until his chest and belly were a mass of red streaks and threads of tissue, his forehead damp in the heat, his bright, alert eyes peppering us with questions and stories. He loved his work, you could see it, he loved the razor in his hand and the heat, the faint coppery odor of blood.

He'd just read an article in *The New Yorker*, and it had drawn him in. The pilots were in their seats, he said, with nuclear bombs armed and ready. The Pakistanis, poised for the Indian cities, Delhi and Calcutta. Fire like you've never seen. One telephone call.

"I am become death, destroyer of worlds," Dr. Whistler said, stretching. "Source?"

"J. Robert Oppenheimer," I replied, "after the Trinity site test."

"Right," he snapped. "And his source?"

"The *Bhagavad Gita*."

"Right again. And which god was he quoting?"

"Shiva," I replied. "He was quoting Shiva."

Dr. Whistler looked at me for a long moment, then nodded. He seemed lost in thought, as if for an instant he'd forgotten where he was. But then he was back.

"Good," he said, looking down to where Mr. Stone's skinned feet lay waiting. "This should do it."

THE SECRET

"YOU HAVE TO COME AND SEE THIS," THE NURSE SAID
breathlessly, interrupting rounds. "It's the grossest thing I ever
saw."

It was early on Sunday morning, and the trauma team had
been shuffling around the surgical ICU for an hour, trying to
impose some order on the carnage of the night before. It was a
blur for me by then, a stream of wounds and bodies. There had
been only two surgery residents and me, and we had been
going for twenty-four hours straight, trying not to miss something big. I felt jumpy, distant from the world, and the bright
white coats and accusing fingers of the surgery attendings
seemed like the fixtures of dreams. I heard myself answering
questions, searching my note cards, I felt numbers emerging
from my mouth, but I wasn't really there. I could smell the odor

of my body rising from my scrubs, and my feet felt loose and wet in my running shoes. But she got my attention anyway. She got everybody's. The grossest thing she ever saw—

Her patient lay in his darkened room, heavily sedated on the ventilator. After two weeks he was getting better, and for the past few days we had virtually ignored him. A young man, drunk, in his car, the same story again, coming slowly back into the world.

"Watch," the nurse said, lifting the flashlight from the bedclothes. We gathered around the bed. With her left hand she moved the clear plastic ventilator tube to the side of the man's mouth, then carefully inserted her fingers between his front teeth and spread them apart. His jaw opened slackly, and she shone the light directly into his mouth.

His mouth was like a little pink cave. Inside were dozens of tiny white worms. As we watched, they began to move, to retreat into the darker recesses, away from the light, and in a few seconds they were gone. "Oh my God," one of the residents said. "They're maggots. He's got maggots in his mouth."

The room erupted. We were horrified, but also excited, exhaustion washed away. He was alive, and we made her do it again. We took turns, switching off the light for a minute or two until the maggots came back, then illuminating them, transfixed by their retreat into the dark.

"What we need to do," Dr. Whistler said, chortling, "is get a piece of bacon on a string and leave it in his mouth for a while. I've seen this before. This is why we don't like flies in the ICU."

One of the medical students went down to the cafeteria for the bacon, and before long the news had spread throughout the hospital. Nurses and medical students and residents from other services began filing through his room until finally the charge nurse put a stop to it. "This isn't a sideshow," she said, to settle the matter.

Tied to a string, raw and shiny with fat, the bacon worked beautifully. The nurse pulled it out every half hour or so, and each time it was alive with maggots. She wiped them off, dropped them into a bottle of alcohol, then replaced the bacon. "It's like fishing," she said, chuckling, shaking her head.

A month or so later, in the trauma clinic, I saw him again, stiff, thin, walking slowly with his cane. The nurse called his name, and he came slowly forward to the desk. We sat a few feet away, and as he stood writing his name on the forms, weak and alive, we whispered.

"That's the maggot man. Remember him? He's right over there."

No one had told him a thing.

SPEAKING IN TONGUES

RUTH WAS A SMALL BRITISH WOMAN WITH CLOSE-CROPPED blond hair and a tiny white triangular scar that lifted the corner of her upper lip just enough to make her look secretly amused. She was the new attending neurosurgeon, already in her early forties, though you wouldn't know it to look at her, with her smooth fair skin, her quick exact movements.

Usually she was calm and polite, but you could never tell what would set her off. Her face would grow still, she would step up close, white-lipped, and empty her flat gray eyes into yours. It didn't matter if her tone was mild, or even if her anger was reasonable; you felt as if a door to a room you did not want to enter had opened, and then closed again.

She was technically skilled, there was no question. She was quick and accurate, and could pop a pressure monitor into the brain in her sleep, her small hands deft on the instruments. But by the end of the year the wards were full of rumors, and she was gone.

Once, in the middle of the night, I brought her a CAT scan to read. She was alone with the scrub nurse in the OR, the anesthetist invisible behind the drapes. Music was playing— chants, a vaguely Cajun rhythm, and I saw, looking in the hollow where her neck rose out of the gown, that she was wearing a black, tie-dyed T-shirt under her scrubs.

A man lay on the table, his head wrapped in sterile plastic. Through a little round hole in the center of his skull, I could see the dura, the thin connective tissue that covers the brain. The dura was a vague blue, bulging, under pressure, and hair, shorn from the man's scalp, lay in brown clumps on the floor by Ruth's feet.

"Thank you, Dr. Huyler," she said, as I came into the room and clipped the scan onto the luminous board. She craned her neck, reading it. "Good. The ventricles are open."

I turned to go, but she stopped me. "Dr. Huyler," she said. "Come here. I want to show you something." I stepped up behind her, careful not to violate the sterile field, and looked over her shoulder at the wound.

"Have you ever seen the movie *Alien*?" She was smiling a little.

"I have."

"Are you familiar with the scene where the alien bursts from the man's chest? On the spaceship?"

"Sure."

"Watch." And she touched the tip of the scalpel to the dura, as delicate as a brushstroke.

At first nothing happened. Then, slowly, a little blue-red worm of drying blood began twisting from the slit like toothpaste, and suddenly the clot spurted out of the man's head like a plum, dripped down past his ear to the drapes.

"That," Ruth said, "is how you take out a subdural hematoma."

WHEN I WAS A BOY my family lived in Brazil, and during those months, as Ruth revealed herself to us, it kept coming back to me—festival night, down by the lake. Ash Wednesday and Africa combined, macumba, or *santería*, or voodoo, call it what you will. The poor gathered there by the hundreds after dark. It was luck they were after, good fortune for the coming year. They stood in the shallows at the water's edge with tiny boats they had made. On the boats were candles, photographs of dead loved ones and saints, offerings: bananas, small pieces of meat, feathers. They said prayers, then pushed the boats into the darkness. If the boats continued out in the water it meant the offerings were accepted. If they returned to shore it meant an indifferent future.

And so nothing was left to chance. The boats were wired, with small electric motors and batteries—expensive in the slums—and they continued, for hundreds of yards, until it was a lake of candles, a small constellation of human need.

A thousand miles to the east, the scene repeated itself on a massive scale, as enormous crowds gathered at the beaches of Rio and Bahia, and the boats went into the open sea. But the people here were too poor to travel, and so they made do with what they had: a small lake, with garbage on the shore, on the outskirts of the inland city. That night, in the dark, it seemed sufficient, beautiful, and the lake vast, without visible edges, full of candles entering the distance until they burned out.

A few yards offshore, hip-deep in the lake in a long line, stood the frogmen of the military police. They stood quietly, their black scuba tanks and wetsuits glittering in the lights off the beach, careful to let the boats pass untouched between them.

ONE NIGHT IN THE ER, as the faint siren of the ambulance grew nearer, I sat with Angela at the doctors' station. She was a surgery resident who had just rotated off the neurosurgery service, and we talked about Ruth. It wasn't my case, I didn't have to go into the trauma room this time, and I felt calm, even content, as I watched. Ruth stood just outside the trauma room, and she was angry again—I could see it in her stiffness as she waited for the ambulance. Someone had called her too soon, before the patient had arrived.

The ER was full, as always, and a man was yelling nearby, his voice heavy and incoherent, that they were hurting him. "It wouldn't hurt if you didn't fight us," a nurse said, breathing hard, as they struggled to hold the man down on the gurney, buckling the leather straps to his wrists and ankles. He was wild, drunk, full of half-formed words, watched by the patients who sat waiting around us.

"I don't know how you work down here," Angela said. The man heaved and bucked on the gurney, and nurses converged, a knot of dark blue scrubs bending over him, until he was quiet. I shrugged my shoulders, and we turned back to Ruth.

Of all of us, Angela knew Ruth the best. By coincidence they had come from the same hospital in Miami, Ruth as a new attending, Angela to complete the last year of her surgery residency. But there was no loyalty between them. "She got really friendly in Miami a couple of years ago," she said, nodding to where Ruth stood down the hall, "when she found out I was from Panama. She said they have some powerful magic down there. It was weird. She invited me over for dinner once and then we went out drinking. Now she acts like she doesn't know who I am."

"She is good, though," she added. "She knows what she's doing." And she was. I remembered, that night before the harvest, the liver transplant, how the pressure monitor had seemed to flow into the young woman's head through Ruth's hands, deep into the ventricle of the brain. And as the numbers climbed on the screen—40, 50, 60—Ruth had shaken her head.

"She'll die," she'd said. "Her intercranial pressure is far too high this early." And then she'd gone off to find the family.

THE FROGMEN WERE THERE for a reason; there had been drownings in the past. Earlier, as I stood in the crowd with my father and mother, watching the boats, I had noticed the women, dressed in white, their black arms dipped in flour. A dozen or so, and even at first they had seemed odd, a strange look in their eyes as they stood near the water. Slowly, one by one, they began to rock, back and forth, murmuring at first, letting it build up in them. Then it would start, the speaking in tongues, the jerking of their bodies as the crowd gathered around them, the convulsing on the ground, and finally, the rush for the lake. They would flip and heave into the shallows, driven out from the beach, soaked dresses clinging to their backs, to their breasts and legs, trying for deeper water. And then the frogmen would converge. It was the moment they had been waiting for, grabbing the women in their arms, picking them up, and dragging them back to the beach. Then the line of divers would reform, and the women would lie back, spent, in the blankets of the crowd until it came on again. It was the force of order, of military rule, against the spirit world: soldiers, with women in their arms, carrying them to the safety of dry ground.

"RUTH KEEPS A COMPLETE fetal skeleton in a jar in her bedroom," Angela said. "She took it out and showed it to me. I couldn't believe it. She told me it reminds her of why she's a surgeon." Angela looked uneasily away, but after a bit she continued, as if talking to herself alone. "Do you know what she did every chance she got when we were in Miami?" I said nothing.

"She'd go to raves. She talks like someone in Masterpiece Theatre, and she was a regular rave-queen. She'd go when she was on call. She'd carry her beeper, and whenever there was a bad head she'd come in smelling of incense. Everyone knew it.

"When we went out that time she got pretty drunk. We were sitting there in this bar, and this middle-aged woman walked by. Ruth was staring at her, I mean, just staring. And then she turns to me. 'Angela,' she says, 'there's something I want to tell you.' 'What,' I say. And then she looks at me, and she whispers, so quiet I can barely hear her. *'I'll fuck anything.'* That was what she said. *'I'll fuck anything.'* I'm telling you, I went home pretty quick."

THE WOMAN CALLED 911, and told the paramedics, very clearly, that she wished to be transported to University Hospital, where her lover was a doctor.

She was big and black, with silver studs running up the arc of her left ear, and she was crying. Her face was a mass of bruises, a split lip, one eye swollen shut, with scratches on her neck.

"Ruth did this to me," the woman said clearly, to anyone who would listen. "Ruth. Ruth did this. This is what she does to me."

But despite all the talk Ruth was the same. She continued, distant and controlled, just as she had been, nodding politely to me in the hall when we passed, a small woman, with small quick steps. They drove her hard, beyond herself. All of us were used to call, to being up thirty-six hours or longer, but as a junior attending Ruth was on call every night, at home with her beeper. On a bad string, if events aligned, she could go for the better part of a week with only scraps of sleep, so tired she could barely stand, until the heads lay shaved beneath her fingers, and she had to do it again.

And then there was that curious phrase, that I heard only once, under her breath, when things were going badly one night: "Esmeralda's going to die tonight."

WHEN ANGELA FINALLY turned Ruth in, the chairman of surgery came into the clinic with a nurse, and they took Ruth with them to the bathroom. As the chairman waited outside, Ruth did what they asked, went into the stall, urinated into the plastic cup while the nurse stood and watched. Of course she knew then that she was finished, but she went back to the clinic anyway, the nurse said, and kept seeing patients as if nothing had happened.

Her urine lit up. Fentanyl. Cocaine. Valium. Marijuana. The drugs of the hospital and the street, and she was gone, the very next day, the headlines—BRAIN SURGEON SHOOTING UP BETWEEN OPERATIONS—suppressed from the city papers. They handled it well—rehabilitation, a special program in another state, paid for by the hospital. No talk. The next plane out.

THREE MONTHS LATER, they rolled the man in, and this time it was mine, this time I couldn't watch from a distance. He was in his fifties, in a suit, ejected from the car, intubated already by the paramedics, and his head, the bones of his skull, felt loose, like gravel and warm bread.

"Call neurosurgery," I said to the nurse, then continued, listening to his chest, feeling his belly, watching the scissors go through the suit cloth as we stripped him.

And then Ruth walked in through the door like a ghost. She was done with rehab, and they'd let her come back. "What do you have for me, Dr. Huyler?" she asked, looking down at the dying man. I stared at her, unable to answer for a few seconds.

"Um, unstable skull fractures. And he's posturing." As I spoke, the man's arms curled again up to his chest, his wrists twisting outward in the darkest of involuntary reflexes. A bad head. His arms had their own intention, their own power, and the nurses struggled to keep the IVs in place.

"OK," Ruth said. "Paralyze him." So I gave the order, the drugs flowed, and he went slack like a dead man.

Ruth had changed, it was as if life had gone from her. She looked tremulous, frail, her skin wrinkled and dry. She looked her true age, she looked uncovered, with none of the strength I was used to, the well I had seen her call on again and again. She was a husk, and as we waited for the CAT scan I tried to make small talk. "Good to have you back," I said, watching her closely. Even then I knew it was a taunt, a match held up to the birdcage, where the hawk sat on a stick.

She looked back at me over the man's still figure, her eyes glittering, and inclined her head. It was the last time I saw her. A few days later they caught her again, and fired her for good.

"She'd been through rehab before," Angela said, "back in Miami, only nobody out here knew about it. Why would it work this time?" I wondered if Angela was afraid now. She showed no sign of it, but she had reason. Ruth's career was over, all those years of work, and she had Angela to blame. "I felt bad about telling on her until her girlfriend called me up. She thanked me for turning Ruth in."

"She *thanked* you?"

Angela nodded. "She told me a lot about Ruth. How every morning before work she'd drink a cup of black coffee and do two lines of coke. Every morning. How when she'd had a really bad day she'd go to the farmers' market and buy a live chicken. She'd take it home and light candles and put on music and cut the chicken's throat with a straight razor."

Esmeralda's going to die tonight.

BUT THE MONTHS PASSED, and Ruth was well and truly gone. No one knew where. Probably she left the city, drifted to the raves of New Orleans or LA, where no one would know who she was. But I'm not certain, and half of me expects to see her again, there in the doorway as I stand by the gurney.

"What do you have for me, Dr. Huyler?" she'll ask, full of prayers and cocaine, smelling like candles. And I'll answer her.

"Gunshot wound," I'll say. "To the head."

POWER

I'M HARD ON HIM, I DON'T GIVE HIM ANY TIME TO PLAN. I have him on the gurney, and his eyes are flicking back and forth. He wants escape, to rise and flee, but he can't. So he starts to cry, and I go right through his tears, purposeful, head down.

"You need it, Mr. Hyde. We're going to put it in whether you like it or not."

"I want my wife!" he cries. "I want my wife."

He is alert from the car; he remembers the crash exactly.

"Can't you do something else? Isn't there another way?"

I say nothing. I'm thinking, there's no other way because this is serious. There is no time to negotiate. It's going in because I think you have a ruptured spleen, and afterward I'm going to stick a needle in that smooth white belly of yours and see. But first we have to put it in, and before that I have to check the prostate.

"Don't put it in, don't put it in, don't do it. Mary! Mary!"

I just nod to the techs, and they grab his legs and spread them apart. "I was abused as a child. I was raped. You don't understand."

I suspected it, and I pause, but it doesn't matter if I understand. You're fifty years old and I think you have a ruptured spleen, and you're going to die unless we know.

"I'm sorry, Mr. Hyde."

"It's not the needle," he gasps to the nurse, "the needle doesn't bother me—"

But I put two gloves on my right hand, lubricate the index finger, and go inside him before he can think.

"Oh, oh, oh!" he cries, but I've done it and peeled off the glove, and it looks OK.

"All right," I say to the techs. They are strong men.

"I don't care if I'm bleeding inside. I don't care. Mary, Mary, no, don't let them, Mary—"

And then he stops speaking, he just goes somewhere else, he vanishes. His face is a great distance. The tech eases the catheter in deep, smooth and quiet, until the urine flows out like gold, and the bladder drains until it's out of the way and safe from the needle.

I wash his belly with iodine, quickly. Then I pop the needle in, just below the belly button, and—Oh, look at this. Do you see what I have in my hand? The syringe is full of blood; your belly is full of blood, I was right, I have a nose for it.

"Mr. Hyde," I say, "you need an operation. We're going to take you upstairs to the operating room right now."

He nods, he sounds like a little boy, his face creases up again, he opens his eyes.

"Do what you want to," he says.

Discharged, five days later, in good condition.

JAW

THE YOUNG WOMAN WAS DRUNK, HER JAW WAS SHATTERED, and as she screamed the air around her head filled with a fine blood mist that beaded up on my goggles and mask. Another car crash, another steering wheel to the chin, but even from the first we knew it wasn't that bad.

"Bobby," she screamed. "Bobby." Bobby was her boyfriend. He lay in the next room, drunk also, with a face full of glass, but just as lucky. As she opened her mouth to scream again, deaf to us, we saw the jagged fracture, the splinter of white bone sticking out from her lower gum.

"Well, one thing's for sure," Rosa said, her eyes shiny, looking up at me.

"What's that?"

"No blow jobs for Bobby anytime soon."

Rosa was a senior surgery resident, famous for such comments. I laughed out loud, and then all of us—Rosa, the techs, the nurses, the intern, and I—just gave in to it. It was terrible, it was grotesque and monstrous, and that made it all the funnier. Tears came to my eyes, ran down my cheeks behind the mask, and through it all the woman screamed, until the morphine eased into her and she went quiet.

Rosa was a short woman, thin, in her late thirties now, brown-eyed, with thin black hair that fell to her shoulders, and coffee-stained teeth. Hers was a tight intelligence, quick and dark, and she used it all the time. She used it on the nurses, she used it on me, and she used it on herself. It was excoriating, sexual, utterly unapologetic.

"Just shut the fuck up," she would yell into the faces of the drunks in the trauma room, pointing at them with a finger. And Dr. MacGregor, the grim chairman of surgery, would shake his head and allow himself a little smile. "Rosa," he'd say, "is a pistol." And then he'd reach out, clap her on the back.

Rosa treated the men under her with a delicate combination of autocracy and desire. She would put her arms around us, rub our backs and thighs, sit down uninvited next to us on the couch of the trauma call room, drape her legs over our laps. "You were great last night, Frank," she'd say, rolling her eyes. "Don't tell me you don't remember."

"Come on, Rosa."

"I can see it coming back. Oh my God, you're thinking, I slept with Rosa. I can't believe it."

And then the change. "What did Ellison's chest X ray from this morning show?"

"No pneumothorax."

"And what else?"

"Nothing else."

"He may have a pneumonia brewing in his right base. I reviewed it with the radiologist. And he's your patient."

"Sorry. I didn't see it." She'd nod and walk away.

She was a terrific surgeon. She knew all the numbers, quick and careful in the OR, standing on a stool so she could see into the field. And in the trauma room she was an absolute presence, curt as the events flowed and unfolded, making her choices. She was in the hospital all the time as the years ticked down, small in her overcoat, crossing through the lights of the parking lot in the early morning, in the evening, back and forth to her bed.

And she ran. I'd see her after call, for miles on the path around the soccer fields. Her face looked drawn, but she kept going in the hot afternoon, fast and lean and tireless. Afterward, she'd climb into her black Jeep, put on her shades, and arrange her hair in the mirror.

When the phone rang one afternoon, I didn't know what to say. "Hi, Frank," she said, sounding uncharacteristically shy. "It's Rosa." We made small talk for a few minutes, and then she got to the point. "Do you want to go to a movie tonight?"

So we sat there in the dark, eating popcorn as the images unrolled above us. I felt her presence strongly, a tingle in my neck and arm, and I realized that in this brief respite of the normal world she had let the chinks in, let the air blow through her. It felt real and human and I went along with it for a little while, in the warmth of the theater, feeling her faintly on my shoulder like static.

I am an average-looking man, thin, with short brown hair and blue eyes. I am faceless in the crowd. I don't think more or less of myself for it. My face betrays nothing in the shaving mirror—no great insight, no great kindness or skill, no contentment or loneliness, no hint of vision or dreams. Just an uncertain face, young, pale, with thin dry hair.

But that night I was lonely, and her loneliness felt like a glass against which mine was magnified. The long nights of call, the whirl of the ER, my empty house which waited at the end of it—so I went along, out of sadness, out of being tired, out of listening to the wind blow through the eaves of my house as I lay down to sleep.

Dinner came next. Pizza, Caesar salad, thick red wine. Hospital talk. Dr. Whistler. Ruth. Dr. Blake. Nurses. Ourselves. "You know," she said, "take Whistler for example. When you first meet him you think, 'what an interesting, kind, intelligent person.' Then after about a week you realize." I nodded. "Or," she continued, "take Blake. He actually had a psychiatric diagnosis. I'm telling you, it really makes me wonder why I'm doing this. I thought I'd be married with kids by now like my sister."

"Oh, come on Rosa," I replied. "You love this stuff and you know it. You thrive on it."

It was the answer she expected, needed, and she smiled, looked down at her plate and the small portion of food that lay there. "I know," she said. "I have the best job in the hospital. It just comes with the worst hours. I signed up, so too bad."

Too bad, I thought, looking at her across the table. She might have been kind, in another life, but she wasn't, at least right now, and neither was I. There was cruelty in us both, as we took turns with the incompetent anesthesia residents, the lesbian gynecologists, the pathetic surgeon drunk on rounds. We were after weakness, real or otherwise, and there was a grim joy in our voices, a kind of complicity, as if we were letting each other in on a rare secret.

"You know," she said, after a while. "It does change us. There's no doubt about it. We'll never be exactly the same."

"You're right," I replied. "No blow jobs for Bobby anytime soon." And we both laughed at that image again, the young woman with a mouthful of bone splinters, spitting blood out onto her chest.

"How did she do, anyway?" I asked.

"Oh, fine," she said. "ENT fixed her jaw and we sent her home."

When the check came she pounced on it. "Why don't you let me pay half?" I asked, a little drunk now.

"Nah," she said. "My treat. You can pay next time."

I thanked her, and as we stood for a few moments on the cold sidewalk outside the restaurant, buttoning our coats, the silence came on. A time for signals, and as I watched her realize that none were coming I knew exactly how she felt. But I kept my face blank and smiling until she knew for sure and said good night, walked the short distance to where her Jeep glittered under the lamp, got in, started the engine, drifted away into the swarm of taillights on the avenue.

As I turned and walked toward my car, I felt empty, a great wash of loneliness coming up from the alleys and shadows, from the interiors of parked cars, from the vague, irregular sky overhead. I didn't feel wanted, or unwanted, worthy, or unworthy. I felt no real pity for her or for myself, no anger, no compassion, just this vacancy, this spending cold.

THE VIRGIN

SHE WAS SO BEAUTIFUL SHE CAUGHT ME. I ENTERED THE
room looking down at her chart, so when I raised my eyes I
had no warning, no time to prepare myself. She was fifteen,
and I was exactly twice her age. But I couldn't help it. She
was oracular, the kind that leaps from the crowd. And she
was used to it, I could tell, but she was shy anyway, and
smiled a small embarrassed smile when she saw me.

A young man stood next to the examination table. He was
older, in his early twenties, and he looked rough. He wore a
black Raiders shirt, baggy jeans, basketball shoes, a buzz cut,
the endless uniform of the gangs, and he stood there staring
with his dark eyes—bird-dogging me, as he would call it. A
challenge, the kind that in the city led to trouble.

"Hello," I said, in my mildest voice. "What can I do for
you?"

"I'm having this itching." She spoke softly. "It itches real bad."

"Where is it?"

"It's down there," she said, not meeting my eye.

"How long have you had it?"

"For two days. It itches real bad."

"It's OK. You can talk about it."

"I don't know what it is."

"When was your last period?"

She started to blush then, beginning in her cheeks and spreading down to her neck, like water flowing out on a table. She glanced at her boyfriend, then back to me. "Does he have to hear?"

"No," I said, looking directly at him, meeting his eye. "If you want him to leave he will."

His face narrowed, and he turned to her. "Do you want me to go?"

"If it's all right," she said, looking at his feet. "I'm embarrassed."

He nodded, shortly, gave me a look, then stepped past and left the room. "I'll be right outside," he said on the way out. "You yell and I'll be there."

A look of relief passed over her face. "I'm sorry," she said. "He gets wild sometimes."

"He's in a gang, right?" As soon as I said it I regretted it. Too far, I thought. She didn't answer directly.

"He won't let me go anywhere without him," she said. "He's always with me." From the tone of her voice I realized that she was proud that he never left her, that he never let anyone look at her, proud that she was his. So I left it alone.

"When was your last period?"

"I'm late," she said quickly, as if to get through it. "I'm two weeks late. That's really why I came here. I don't want him to know."

"We'll do a pregnancy test. Is there anything else? Have you noticed any discharge?"

"Discharge?"

"Stuff coming out? A bad smell?"

"Well"—she looked suddenly her age, and afraid—"I guess so."

"All right. I'll tell you what we need to do. I need you to pee in this cup, and then I'll come in with the nurse and do a pelvic exam. Have you had one of those before?"

She shook her head slowly. "I don't think so."

"OK. It's not so bad. I'll come back in a few minutes with the nurse and we'll explain it." She nodded, and I left the room. Outside, in the hall, her boyfriend lay sprawled on one of the spare gurneys, staring grimly at the ceiling, his arms crossed behind his head. He didn't look at me, or speak, as I passed him.

A moment later the door opened, and she stepped out, clutching the gown to her body. She came tentatively over to the desk where I sat.

"Um, I don't know who I'm supposed to give this to," she said, blushing again as she handed me the jar. It was warm in my hand, gold, full of urine.

"Thanks. I'll give it to the nurse."

With a start I realized that I hadn't told her where the bathroom was, that she had urinated into the cup in her room, crouching down on the floor.

The nurse and I entered the room a few minutes later. "Anna," I began, sitting down on the stool, "here's what we're going to do." And I showed her the speculum, the light, and the swabs. "It may be a bit uncomfortable, but it shouldn't hurt. If it hurts just tell me and I'll stop."

There's no avoiding the power of that moment, what floats out of you like a secret. You just don't acknowledge it. You banish it with an act of will. You are breezy, conversational. She's fifteen years old, and she's crying, and the nurse is holding her hand like her mother, but she's beautiful anyway, and you feel dark, ashamed, you do not like what you see in yourself. By then you're inside, you open the speculum, and it looks fine, and then you flick in the swabs and you're done.

"Everything looks normal, Anna. There's just one more thing." I stood up close, between her ankles, feeling her uterus and ovaries. They were firm, like knots, and small, as they should have been. "There, Anna. We're done. You did great. Everything looks fine."

And so she sat up, wiping her eyes with the back of her hand. "I don't want my mom to find out," she said. "Don't tell my mom."

"Don't worry, Anna. We won't tell your mom. No one will know." And with that I left the room, carried the test tube to the lab in the back, wiped the swab on the microscope slide, adjusted the lenses, and they came swimming up. Cells, normal epithelium, and what I suspected: clear little tendrils, with buds. Yeast.

"Anna," I said, coming back into the room. "Your pregnancy test was negative, but you have a yeast infection. I'll give you some medicine for it and it should go away in a few days." Her face softened, she opened her eyes and smiled, looking right at me.

"Thank you," she said, and she looked so happy that I felt old. As she stood in the hallway with her boyfriend, putting on her coat, smiling delightedly at him as he tapped his foot and scowled, I thought of what I'd also seen on the slide. Dead, like calligraphy, like dozens of little sticks twirling slowly beneath the lens. Sperm.

SUGAR

THE LITTLE GIRL WAS RUNNING AROUND THE ROOM, screeching happily, and when she saw me she hid under the bed. I could see her peering at me from between the legs of the gurney as I stood with her chart in my hand. Her father shook his head, grinned, and looked at his wife. "I told you there's nothing wrong with her."

I looked down at the chart. On it the triage nurse had written, in bold black letters, "Two-year-old acting weird."

"I'm Dr. Huyler," I said. "What can I do for you?"

"Nothing," the man said, and his wife hushed him.

"She's not acting right," she said. She wore an African print dress, and I found myself staring at the intricate pattern of swirling reds and browns. Her hair was cornrowed, a bead at the end of each strand.

"They're Medicaid," the triage nurse had whispered pointedly in my ear. The implication was clear: they wanted something for free. Tylenol, a work excuse. But it was ten o'clock on a Friday night.

"What has she been doing?"

"It's kind of hard to explain. She just isn't acting herself. I noticed it right away. But she's been fine ever since we got here."

"Can you be more specific?" I could feel myself getting impatient. There were half a dozen patients waiting, the ER was full. I wondered why they hadn't called their regular pediatrician.

"Well," she said, thinking. "You know how people look when they're staring into a mirror? Kind of blank?" I nodded. "She's like that. Only there isn't a mirror. There's nothing there."

The child's vital signs were completely normal. Her mother coaxed her out from under the bed and held her wriggling in her arms as I listened to her heart and lungs, looked into her ears.

I'm uneasy with children. I must have been a cold, white form to her, large, bending down with my stethoscope and light. I could see nothing wrong with her. She looked impeccably cared for, without any sign of the abuse I had been vaguely and secretly considering. I always do. It's been drummed into us.

"Does she have any medical problems at all?"

"No," her father said, anticipating my questions. "She's always been healthy. She's had all her shots. She's growing like she should, and she can talk a little, only now she won't 'cause she's shy." He wagged a finger, and she giggled, hiding her face with the bottle her mother had given her.

"Has she had any recent stress, something that might have upset her?" They looked at each other.

"I don't think so."

"Is there any history of seizures in the family?"

Her mother thought for a while. "I think my brother might have seizures," she said finally, "but I haven't seen him in a long time."

"And right now she's acting normally?"

"She's fine," her father said to his wife. "Come on, let's go. If she does it again we'll come back. It's past her bedtime."

I considered what I'd heard. A vague history of blank spells; it could mean anything, from a rare type of seizure to the vagaries of the two-year-old mind. She could see her pediatrician on Monday, I thought. She was a completely normal child.

On my way out the door, though, I turned around. "Is there any chance she might have gotten into someone's medications? Does anyone in the family take medications regularly?"

"Well, she stays with my mother when we're at work. She takes medicines."

"What kind of medicine does she take?"

"I'm not sure. Something for her blood pressure and a sugar pill."

Oral hypoglycemics—sugar pills—are among the most dangerous of overdoses. They can drop blood sugar profoundly, cause brain damage, seizures, coma. Designed for adult diabetics, they are long-lasting, and one pill could kill a small child, even many hours later.

"Let's check her blood sugar," I said, "just to be sure. And please call your mother, find out exactly what she takes."

From the doctors' station I could hear the child shrieking as the nurse drew her blood. Her mother spoke into the phone a few feet away.

"My mother takes glipizide," she said, handing me a piece of paper where she'd written it down. "She ran out of her blood pressure medicine two weeks ago."

A sugar pill.

The nurse came out of the room with a syringe full of blood. The child's mother and I watched as she eased a single drop from the tip of the needle onto the portable blood-sugar machine she held in her hand. It digested the blood for a few seconds, then displayed the number on the screen. Forty-two.

"Is that low?" her mother asked.

"It's about half of what it should be," I replied, stunned. "She must have taken one of your mother's sugar pills."

"My mother is legally blind. She probably dropped one and didn't notice."

"We need to keep her in the hospital for at least a day and give her sugar intravenously." I said it quietly, half to myself.

"Will she be all right?" She was afraid, staring at me. "She'll be fine." And suddenly I began to shake. "But I'm very glad you brought her in. You may have saved her life."

"My husband wanted to put her to bed," she said softly, looking off down the hall.

It was suddenly clear. Sometime that afternoon the girl had taken the pill, and by the time her parents came home she was showing the effects of low blood sugar: the staring spells, the blank look.

"What did you do when you saw she was acting weird?"

"We gave her a bottle," the father said, standing with us now. "And then we gave her a sucker."

They had given her sugar. When she arrived in the ER her blood sugar had risen enough for her to look and act herself, but it wouldn't have lasted long. Later that night, when the whole family was asleep, it would have fallen again, and she might never have woken up.

As I watched the girl skip and jump around us, the pain of the needle forgotten already, I felt sick, cold, and damp, terrified by what I had almost missed. One question, an afterthought. That was all it had been.

From time to time I think about her. I imagine her playing in parks, jumping on the couch, shrieking in the bathtub. I imagine her head teeming with small thoughts, and the motion of her hands, her eyes, alive in the world, going out into it, entering it, decade after decade ahead.

LIAR

SHE LAY THERE AND WOULDN'T TALK TO ME, STARING AT the ceiling with her pale blue eyes. I felt myself getting angry. "I can't talk," she mouthed, as if to a lip-reader.

I knew she was lying. "You can talk," I said. "Why don't you tell me what's wrong?"

She mouthed some more, and I started, despite myself, to hate her. I am complex, she said. I am so complicated, so interesting. Look, you see—I can't talk at all. She was sixty years old, and lay still on the gurney, full of trickery. So I moved closer, pressed my stethoscope against her thin gray chest.

"Ow," she cried, suddenly, in a loud voice. "You're hurting me."

"So you can talk," I replied. She merely looked at the ceiling.

"You don't have to be rude," she said, after a while. "You don't have to be rude to me."

"Why don't you tell me what's wrong?"

"I fell. I fell and hit my head."

Normal vital signs. Now she was silent again. No bruises, not a mark on her. Just her unblinking eyes, looking straight up. Thin, old, wizened. From out of town. Her eyes glittered, fixed on the ceiling. "Did you take any pills? Have you taken anything?"

She shook her head. "I fell," she whispered. "Yesterday." She'd walked into the ER. She moved her arms and legs, but whenever I touched her, even in the slightest way, she cried out. And back at the desk, I heard her howling as the nurses started the IV.

Where to begin? Blood work, a CAT scan of her head. Maybe something would show up, something I could use to get her admitted and out of the ER. She'd exhausted me already.

Her daughter-in-law arrived late, a thin woman with permed gray hair and large, owlish glasses. "I think she fell, yesterday," she said. Then she added in a conspiratorial whisper, "She drinks. She keeps wine in her room." I nodded, ordered some more tests: a blood alcohol level, a tox screen. Thyroid functions. An erythrocyte sedimentation rate. Clever, I thought to myself.

Then her doctor, long distance from New York. "She's a hard one," he said, cheerfully. "She's got a long psychiatric history, she malingers, she drinks, she takes pills when she can get them. Good luck." As I sat talking to him, I could see her lying motionless on the gurney, ignoring the psychiatrist who stood next to her and tried to ask her questions.

The psychiatrist shook his head when he came out of the room. "She won't talk to me," he said. "She's completely uncooperative."

I called medicine, and medicine came down. "Her CAT scan was normal," I said. "All of her blood work is normal. She has normal vital signs. She's not drunk. She has a psych history. She won't talk to me or to the psychiatrist. I'd like to see what you think."

"Thank you," medicine replied, rolling her eyes, "for this interesting consult." She was still in there, examining the woman, when I left.

As I drove home, fast on the interstate, past the dark snow-covered fields, I couldn't get her out of my mind. She was a mystery. I should have done a spinal tap, I told myself. I should have looked at her spinal fluid. Meningitis, I thought. Or encephalitis. And I had considered it. But I simply hadn't wanted to hold her down, to curl her into a ball on her side and pop the needle into her gritty, arthritic back as she howled and writhed. She bothered me, though, and when I got home I called the ER. "What did you do with her?"

"I sent her home. The minute I started talking about the spinal tap she got a lot more cooperative."

Weeks passed, a month. I still thought about her, about her infuriating gaze, lying to me, sad though I couldn't feel it. Not really. A sponge, an absorber of energy and time, for unclear useless ends.

On Saturday morning, the nurse from risk management

was waiting for me. "There's a doctor in New York who wants to talk to you," she said. "About a patient you saw. Here's his number." And she handed me the chart. There she was. A fall? Uncooperative. Normal labs and vitals. And then the discharge diagnosis: headache of unclear etiology. Not a mark on her.

The doctor, when I reached him, was a storyteller. And a neurosurgeon. "What happened?" I could feel my voice rising. He came through clearly on the cell phone, driving home from the city.

"Well," he said, slowly. He wasn't going to let me off easy. "After she saw you, she stayed in town for two more weeks. Walking around. Then she got on the plane to come back to New York." I waited.

"Apparently she started screaming on the plane. She screamed so much that they landed the plane in Dallas and took her off by ambulance to an ER there. They didn't know what to make of her, and I gather they watched her for a few hours and then sent her out. She got back on the plane, made it back here, and then she called up her doctor."

"That's Dr. White?" The man I'd spoken with, a month ago now.

"That's right. Well, he didn't really know what to do with her either. He says she was complaining of a headache. So a few days later she called me. I got some X rays because I thought she might have arthritis in her cervical spine."

He paused. "Come on," I said. "What does she have?"

"She has," he replied, measuring the effect, "the worst broken neck I've ever seen in someone who wasn't paralyzed or dead."

A hangman's fracture occurs when the neck is extended suddenly and violently backward. The second cervical vertebra cracks in half. When the hangman does his job, and reads the chart correctly, and matches the length of the rope to the body weight, the snap at the end of the fall crushes the spinal cord and paralyzes the body. Consciousness is lost only when blood stops flowing to the brain. It takes a few seconds; hanging, even in the best of hands, is not as quick an end as it seems.

That was what she had. The fall must have thrown her head back. It was as if she'd been cut down from the scaffold after the job had been botched. And she'd walked around like that for weeks, when the slightest fall, even a quick jerk, might have finished her.

"How's she doing?" I heard myself ask.

"Amazingly well," he said. "She was so osteoporotic the bones in her neck were like putty. The wires pulled right through. So I just straightened her out and put her in traction. She's completely intact."

Completely intact—no nerve damage, not even a tingle. I could see her lying there in the steel halo, with screws in her temples and a weight, her blue eyes open to the ceiling. Gray hair, a thin face, and her voice, her victorious little whisper, stretched out on the rack: "I can't talk. I just can't talk at all."

THE BEE STING

THE NURSE CAME UP TO ME. "THE GUY IN FOUR WANTS antibiotics for his sore throat. Can I give him something?"

I glanced at his chart. He had a cold, that was all, and it was busy. "I haven't even seen him yet," I said.

The nurse rolled her eyes. "He's just going to keep bugging me."

The ER was full, it was the middle of the night, and I was feeling sorry for myself. Yesterday they had slept.

The waiting room was full of children. Coughs, runny noses, fevers, keeping their parents up until they'd had enough. I'd seen the look so many times—the worn-out mother, the whimpering child whom I would simply send home again. See your pediatrician in the morning. Give him some Tylenol and lots of juice.

Nothing bad was happening, it was all stuff I could bang out in my sleep. Penicillin for the ears. Cough drops and fluids. If he gets worse bring him back.

After a while you come to rely, more than anything else, on first sight. You walk into the room and you think, sick or not sick. Not sick goes home as fast as possible. Sick, you watch. You draw blood, you order X rays, you give them fluids. You are careful, because a little bell went off when you walked into the room and saw them. The nurses do it, too, and when they say, "I don't like how this kid looks," you really pay attention if you're smart. It's something you either learn or you don't. Sometimes I think I've learned it. Sometimes not.

The man in four was not sick. He had a cold and couldn't sleep. It was two in the morning, he shouldn't have been there, and the waiting room looked like a school yard. The nurse came up to me again. "The guy in four wants something for his throat. He keeps bugging me."

"I'll be there in a minute. Tell him to wait."

The man lying on the bed looked perfectly healthy. He was in his early thirties, fat, with curly black hair, a runny nose, and small rectangular eyeglasses. On the off-chance that he had strep throat, I knew that I would give him an antibiotic. But it was a virus.

"You have a sore throat?"

"Yes, it's terrible. I can't sleep. I'm congested. I've had it for a week." His throat was red, his tonsils angry and swollen, lit up by my penlight.

"Are you allergic to any medications?"

"I think I'm allergic to penicillin and erythromycin. You should ask my mom."

"Are you allergic to Keflex?"

"I don't think so. Ask my mom. She's outside somewhere."

"I'm asking you."

"Whatever," he said. "Just give me something for my throat."

"OK," I said to the nurse as I left the room. "Give him some Keflex now, and get him out of here." He could fill the rest of the prescription in the morning. Even if he were allergic to penicillin, the risk of a reaction to Keflex was slight—less than 10 percent. The charts were piling up in the rack.

Thirty minutes later, as I bent over another child with an earache, holding her head with one hand and the otoscope with the other, as she struggled and cried, they came and got me.

"The patient in four is in respiratory distress."

He sat bolt upright on the bed, wheezing, fighting for air, his fingers and toes darkening, with that look on his face, and I knew right away that I was in for it. There was no one to call, no one to turn to. I was the only doctor in the hospital. "Page X ray and respiratory therapy stat. Give him a milligram of epinephrine sub-Q now. Susan, start a line." He was blue, his eyes wide open and reaching.

"We can't get a line, he's a hard stick."

Commands started flowing out of my mouth, without conscious thought. You and you, work on IVs. You, give him another milligram of epinephrine sub-Q. You, get me a central line kit now. You, put him on a hundred percent face mask with an albuterol nebulizer. All of the nurses were there by then.

When people die of bee stings, this is what kills them. Anaphylaxis, the immune system set off like a bomb, and no one knows exactly why. It's rare; I had never seen a case. The whole body swells into hives, the throat constricts, the lungs spasm and close, the blood pressure falls, and it's over in a few minutes.

I knew what I had to do: get a tube down his throat before it swelled shut, and force the oxygen into him. And then I had to give him drugs, epinephrine, SoluMedrol, Benadryl, albuterol, dopamine. Even then it would be a near thing. But we still had to start an IV.

All of us stuck him with needles until his arms were a mass of puncture wounds, oozing dark blue blood onto the sheets, and finally Carol slid one in.

"Give him 100 milligrams of succinylcholine IV push."

Succinylcholine is a similar to curare. It paralyzes you completely, and this is why the monkeys of South America, hit with a poison dart, fall out of their trees and die. They are awake and alert, but they can't breathe.

There was no choice. He could breathe a little on his own, but not enough. He writhed and fought us on the gurney, he snatched the oxygen from his face, he had lost the ability to reason, and I knew that I could never get the tube down him the way he was. So I paralyzed him.

Even as I gave the order I knew I might not be able to pass the tube into his lungs; his lips and eyes were already swelling. If I couldn't, I had one other chance: last-ditch surgery, a scalpel into the trachea, which I had never done.

The drugs flowed, and he was a still figure, blue, like a body. A sense of resignation settled over me as I put the blade into his mouth, lifted his tongue and jaw. But there they were, like a vision, I could see them, as white as paper, the triangle of the vocal cords, and in a second the tube was in.

Oxygen flowed under pressure. Imperceptible, at first, the change in color, and then it was real, and the blue eased from his face, flowing out of his chest and belly, then out of his arms, the way water dries.

But his blood pressure started to fall.

Open his fluids wide. More epinephrine, start a drip. Get another IV. BP 80/53, heart rate 160.

His mother waited in the consultation room. I walked in and sat down, and for the first time there I was the one shaking, I was the one sick and damp with sweat.

"Mrs. Lopez, I'm very sorry. Your son had a reaction to one of the medicines we gave him. He stopped breathing for a while. He's in critical condition, and I'm sending him by ambulance to the big hospital downtown where they can deal with problems like this." I said it in a rush, barely looking at her.

"This is because of a medicine you gave him?"

I nodded. "He's had a terrible allergic reaction. I was able to bring him back, but I don't know what's going to happen. He might still die."

She looked across the room. "My only son," she said, her lips tightening. "What have you done to my son?"

I sent him, blood pressure next to nothing, by ambulance to the ICU downtown, where the pulmonologists and the intensivists waited, and I stared at the empty cubicle, the trash on the floor from the frenzy of the past minutes, a smear of blood, a piece of IV tubing, alcohol pads, and there in the corner, his glasses, their tiny square lenses shining under the fluorescent lights.

The waiting room was still full of children. I had to see them. I had to go in, to look in their ears and listen, but he filled me completely. I was gone, I was somewhere else.

"Say that again?"

"He started coughing yesterday, and then the fever started. You know, we've been waiting a really long time. Is it always this slow?"

I kept running to the phone.

That morning, at home in my bed, I could not sleep, and I was exhausted. His still figure on the gurney, blue, his open eyes—back and forth and back again. Less than 10 percent. By early afternoon I could stand it no longer, and I called again.

"ICU."

"This is Dr. Huyler. I'm calling about Mr. Lopez. He was admitted early this morning, and I'd like to find out how he's doing."

"I'm sorry, sir, we no longer have a patient here by that name."

"Can you tell me what happened to him?"

"Hold on, I'll get the nurse."

Then the silence of waiting, the seconds streaming past, and at last the nurse's voice. "Yes, Doctor. He was transferred to the subacute unit an hour ago. They're going to take him off the ventilator this evening." I had never wanted anything so much.

The days passed, a first, a second, and by the third day I knew it would be all right. But I had to do one more thing.

His room was on the fifth floor overlooking the city, and the sun lit up the mountains in the distance. It was early in the morning when I entered the room, and I heard his voice. He was standing up, talking on the telephone, the swells of his pale white back falling out of the open hospital gown. He heard me enter, and turned.

It took him a little while. At first, I saw the question on his face, and as it slowly gave way to recognition I realized that he was afraid of me.

"Mr. Lopez."

"Mom, I have to go," he said hurriedly into the phone. "That doctor's here."

"You," he said, then paused. A long silence, and I stood there until he broke it.

"This never should have happened," he said, gathering himself, pointing at me with a thick finger. I heard the anger in his voice, and as I looked at him, nodding as he accused me, humbling myself with an act of will, I felt suddenly large and powerful, somehow proprietary. I had nearly killed him, and then I had brought him back from the edge, I had caught his hand just as he fell into the empty spaces and held him there. His anger sustained me: it meant he was undamaged, it meant that he was safe, nearly home again.

"I'm sorry this happened, Mr. Lopez."

"Easy for you to say," he said, his eyes glittering.

He was so alive.

THE HOUSE IN
THE WILDERNESS

THE MAN LOOKED FAMILIAR, BUT I COULDN'T PLACE HIM.
He sat on the side of the bed, monitor wires leading from
his thin brown chest to the screen. Chest pain, the nurse said,
with a cardiac history.

I introduced myself, and we shook hands. "It's terrible," he
said, "this pressure in my chest. It started two hours ago, and
it's getting worse. It feels exactly like a heart attack."

"You've had a heart attack?"

"I've had three, four if you count this one. And heart surgery
lots of times." His white shirt lay folded on a chair, and next to
it a pair of stainless-steel crutches. His left leg was gone. He
wore a bolo tie, old, heavy, dark with silver and turquoise. It
was beautiful, and as the nurse came in to start the IV I men-
tioned it.

"It was my grandfather's," he said. "It's over a hundred years old."

He lay back, extended his tongue for the nitroglycerin in an easy, practiced motion. Then he yawned luxuriously and looked at his watch. "Ooh, it's late," he said. "My girlfriend is expecting me." He winked at the nurse. "She's almost as beautiful as you."

It was nearly three in the morning, and I looked absently at the blood on my white tennis shoes, fine drops from one of the traumas earlier in the evening. The pace of the emergency room was slowing now.

"I'm feeling short of breath," he said. I looked at him, his chest moving easily, his lungs clear under my stethoscope. His heart sounded normal and steady, each beat a green light on the monitor. Bending close to him, I smelled alcohol on his breath.

"How many heart attacks have you had?"

"I've had three heart attacks, four heart surgeries, six heart catheterizations, and last year they cut off my leg. I had"—he paused, looked intently at me—"have you ever seen boiling tar, poured on the road?"

"Yes, I think I have."

"Do you know how it has those bubbles in it?" I nodded. "That's what my leg looked like." He made an angry chopping motion. "Ah shit," he said. "What's a one-legged man good for?"

"Lots of things," I said vaguely, in the silence that followed. He looked at the nurse, then smiled a forced smile.

"I'm still good for that," he said, reaching out and touching her arm. She shrugged him off.

"Don't be a dirty old man," she said. "Behave yourself."

He rubbed his chest and winced. "She's lucky I'm old," he said to me. Then, "How old are you?"

"I'm thirty-one."

"Pah, that's nothing. You haven't lived at all." And he looked down at his leg.

Mr. Santana had an abnormal EKG. "How bad is it?" he asked, peering intently into my face.

"It's abnormal," I replied, "but I need to see an old EKG for comparison. It may not have changed."

"I've been here lots of times before," he said, "and they always want to put me in the hospital." He ran his hand through his dyed black hair, carefully preserving the part, and suddenly I knew who he was.

"Do you have a house in the Pecos wilderness? With adobe walls?"

He looked at me with astonishment. "How did you know that? How did you know about my house?"

"I've taken care of you before," I said. "A few years ago. You left against my advice. Do you remember?"

He inspected me closely. "I don't know," he said, after a while. "I've seen so many doctors. Was I rude to you?"

"No," I answered. "You were very polite."

"I'm sorry if I was rude. Before my wife died I was rude. Now I'm nice. Isn't that right?" He looked at the nurse.

"You're being nice now," she said. "Let's see how long you can stay nice."

"It's beautiful in the Pecos. No electricity, just candles and a well. Nothing changes, it's always exactly the same. My mother was born there. That's where I want to be buried."

"That's what you said last time. I told you you weren't going to die."

"Well, what do you think now? Am I going to die this time?"

"No," I said. "You're not."

Once again the chart confirmed the story: gangrene, his leg amputated just above the knee. He'd also been to the ER five times in the past year, leaving against advice each time. His EKG had not changed. When I came back to his room he was dressed. "Give me the form," he said. "I'm leaving. You can't help me here."

"I'm sorry you feel that way."

"No offense. I like you. But my girlfriend is expecting me. Please get me the form." He struggled up off the gurney, stood on one leg. "Will you hand me my crutches?" The nurse placed them under his arms. She was gentle, even tender.

"Where is the form?"

He took the pen she handed him, wrote his name with a quick, vigorous flourish. But the ink didn't flow, and he scratched the side of the form until it was clear that the pen was empty.

"Your pen is no good," he said, handing it back to me, immaculate in his white dress shirt, a gold cigarette case darkening the pocket, the empty leg of his pants pinned up to his thigh.

As he walked down the hall, his crutches left tiny gray tracks on the waxed floor.

TIME

SOMETIMES WHEN I CATCH A GLIMPSE OF MYSELF IN A mirror, or reflected in a glass door, I understand why they're surprised when I enter the room. Their eyes widen. They often ask me.

"I'm older than I look," I say, which is true. They're usually about ten years off when they guess.

"Is that the doctor? Really?" This from the twenty-year-old nursing assistants, the X-ray techs who don't know me yet. They smile and shake their heads.

I mind and I don't mind. When they see a kid in front of them, they don't want it or expect it. They want the reassurance of age, the visible sign of experience. What they see disturbs them. They ask themselves, Is it possible?

"I want to take you home with me," one old woman says,

"because you're so sweet." I'm not sweet, though. I'm still and distant, and what she wants to take home is the idea of sweetness. But I play along, and she smiles and holds my hand.

In the morning, I wait for them. They begin to trail in around noon, and then the hours flow by as I move from patient to patient, ordering lab work, listening to chests and feeling bellies, looking in ears, deflecting them. They are angry because they also have to wait. I don't care, not even a little. We're going as quickly as we can, I say. There are lots of sick people here.

Sometimes I'm angry. The kid with the bullet hole through the toe, slick black hair, shades, a thin angular face. Nine-millimeter, a party.

"You're too young to be a doctor."

He's seven years younger than I am, and I ready the needle. I'm going to numb up his toe until it feels like a piece of wood, and then I'm going to open the bullet wound and run a half-gallon of saline through it.

"I know," I say. "I'm kind of nervous. This is the first time I've done this." He blanches, he looks stricken, and I stand back, squirt a jet of clear lidocaine straight up into the air to clear the needle. And I let a moment pass. "Don't worry," I say. "I'm kidding. I'm the attending physician in the emergency room. I've done this lots of times."

He smiles, he shakes his head, we chuckle a little bit. He looks away, and is faceless to me as I squeeze the plunger. The skin at the base of his toe swells and whitens and burns. Then he lets me do what I want.

"Can you feel that?"

"No. I don't feel nothing now." Just as quickly, my anger is gone. A flash.

The nurse comes to the bedside. "There's a patient upstairs to pronounce," she says. "Room ten twenty-five. No rush." Odds whisper around us, wheels turn, molecules whir like bobbins. And then, maybe once or twice in our whole lives, events conspire, statistics align with the force of diamonds against us, and they knock us out, there is no chance, the wind blows through us, we're gone. Sometimes we come back. It's magic and real. Those we love walk in, they sit down at the side of the bed. They hold our hands, they look into our eyes and weep, which is what the body does.

I like them when they are brave in the face of it. I like the old women who say they're ready, that they understand the surgery is dangerous, if they die they die, who smile and pat my hand and tell me to send their children in. I like the men who flirt with the nurses even though the EKG is unmistakable.

In room 1025, the old man's eyes are blue and cold, and I close them. I feel for his pulse, listen to his still heart. Then I look at my watch and write down the time: 2:05 A.M. I sign my name.

When I get back the kid is still there. The anesthesia has worn off.

"Jeez, it's starting to hurt. Can you give me something for the pain?"

"How did you get here? Did you drive?"

"My truck's outside."

"Sorry. I can give you a prescription. But nothing here, if you're going to drive." So I write him for some pills, and he hobbles out on crutches, thin and young and trying to pretend he isn't afraid.

It's late, and I go outside, stand in the entrance by the pneumatic doors, look to where the east lightens. I feel strong, but I know it won't last. The quiet city, slow in the lights. Cars pass down the avenue, one, two, a third. Something moves beside me, startling, and I turn. It's just the nurse, Susan, fumbling with her cigarettes.

"Not a bad night," she says, then adds the obligatory superstition. "So far." I nod and smile, watch the flare of the lighter and then the little coal at the tip of her cigarette, blooming as she takes a deep drag and lets the smoke out into the air. It twirls around us both, and we're quiet.

I'm thirty-two years old.